Exploring Our
Environmental Connections

Exploring Our Environmental Connections

Eleanor A. Schuster and Carolyn L. Brown

Editors

National League for Nursing Press • *New York*
Pub. No 14-2634

Copyright © 1994
National League for Nursing
350 Hudson Street, New York, NY 10014

ISBN 0-88737-628-2

This book was set in Garamond by Publications Development Company, Crockett,
Texas. The editor was Maryan Malone, the designer was Allan Graubard. The
printer was Clarkwood Corp. The cover was designed by Lauren Stevens. The
center cover art is the cover designer's rendition of a photograph by Dr. Barbara
Kazanis, University of South Florida, Tampa, FL.

Printed in the United States of America.

For our Earth
Our love and our life
May we return to her
As it has been given us
Full measure, pressed down and running over
and
for our Beautiful Florida
may her River of Grass always flow
clear and pure*

*To this end, we commit any proceeds we may earn from this book to efforts to preserve The Everglades so it may continue to live that we all may live.

A Note on Authorship

As authors, we wish to acknowledge the path for our authorship of this work and place it in the shifting paradigm of nonhierarchical relationships. We both recall the birth of this work. Eleanor Schuster conceived of and coordinated nursing's first environmental conference, held in Boca Raton, Florida, in March 1993. Carolyn Brown, acting as program coordinator for the conference, worked closely with Eleanor and the rest of the conference planning committee to bring the ideas to life. Often, from a conference like this, where ideas flow, a book is born. When this occurred, Eleanor invited Carolyn to join her as coeditor. This book reflects the new paradigm in work where the traditional hierarchical relationships no longer apply. Carolyn suggested Eleanor be first author/editor because she conceived the idea and because first authorship has meaning in our hierarchy-conscious society. The book, however, reflects respectful work of both editors. We have shared equally in the joys and struggles of bringing this work to life.

E.A.S.
C.L.B.

Contributors

Cathy Appleton, PhD, ARNP, CS
Associate Professor
Interim Graduate Program Director
Florida Atlantic University
College of Nursing
Boca Raton, Florida

Charlotte D. Barry, MSN, RN
Visiting Assistant Professor
Florida Atlantic University
College of Nursing
Boca Raton, Florida

Carolyn L. Brown, PhD, RN
Associate Professor
Director, Nursing Administration Program
Barry University
School of Nursing
Miami Shores, Florida

Margaret A. Burkhardt, PhD, RN
Associate Professor of Nursing
Robert C. Byrd Health Sciences Center
West Virginia University
School of Nursing
Charleston, West Virginia

Sherrilyn Coffman, DNS, RN, CPN
Associate Professor
Florida Atlantic University
College of Nursing
Boca Raton, Florida

Craig A. Cookman, PhD, RN
Assistant Professor
University of Nebraska Medical Center
College of Nursing
Lincoln, Nebraska

Marcia Dombro, MSEd, RN, EdD candidate
Former Director of Nursing Education
Baptist Hospital of Miami
Miami, Florida

Susan Elsom, B.Ed
Lecturer
The Caroline Chisholm School of Nursing
Monash University
Frankston, Victoria, Australia

Joyce C. Kadandara
BA (Hons), Diploma Administration State SRN, SCM
Deputy Secretary, Health Support Services
Ministry of Health and Child Welfare
Causeway, Harare, Zimbabwe

Anie Sanentz Kalayjian, EdD, RN, C, DDL
Private Psychotherapy Practitioner
Secretary/Treasurer, United Nations Committee on Human Rights
New York, New York

Dorothy Kleffel, DNSc, RN
Instructor
Azusa Pacific University
San Diego, California

Dianne Lacroix, RN, BScN, MRCNA
Master Candidate
La Trobe University
Assistant Secretary, Nursing the Environment
Melbourne, Victoria, Australia

Patricia L. Munhall, EdD, ARNP, PsyA, FAAN
Professor and Associate Dean of Graduate Program
Director, Center for Nursing Research
Director, Primary Nursing Center
Barry University
Miami Shores, Florida

Kathleen Musker, MA, RN
Whole Health Options
Chicago, Illinois

Elisabeth A. Pennington, EdD, RN
Dean and Professor
College of Nursing
University of Massachusetts—Dartmouth
North Dartmouth, Massachusetts

Marilyn A. Ray, PhD, RN, CTN, CNAA
Associate Professor
Florida Atlantic University
Boca Raton, Florida

University of Colorado Health Sciences Center
School of Nursing
Denver, Colorado

Yingling Visiting Scholar 1994-95
Medical College of Virginia
Virginia Commonwealth University
Richmond, Virginia

Selina Rwashana
Health Education
Ministry of Health
Entebbe, Kampala, Uganda

Phyllis R. Schultz, PhD, RN
Associate Professor of Nursing
School of Nursing
University of Washington
Seattle, Washington

Robert C. Schultz, PhD
Professor of Philosophy
University of Washington
Bothell, Washington

Eleanor Schuster, DNSc, RN
Associate Professor
Florida Atlantic University
College of Nursing
Boca Raton, Florida

Hollie Shaner, RN, BA
President, CGH Environmental Strategies, Inc.
Burlington, Vermont

Bev Taylor, PhD, RN, RM
Professor
Foundation Chair in Nursing
Southern Cross University
Lismore, New South Wales, Australia

Betsy Todd, MPH, BSN, RN
Adjunct Faculty
Hunter-Bellevue School of Nursing
City University of New York
New York, New York

Jean Watson, PhD, RN, FAAN
Distinguished Professor of Nursing
Director, Center for Human Caring
School of Nursing
University of Colorado Health Sciences Center
Denver, Colorado

Acknowledgments

A project like this has no real beginning and no real end. Much thought and care went into all the work preceding the book, and much will flow from its publication. We are grateful to the many people and organizations providing the help, encouragement, and suggestions necessary to create it. First, we gratefully acknowledge the many chapter contributors. Without their efforts, there would be no book. We are especially grateful to Hazel Henderson, who graciously agreed to write the foreword. The Florida Atlantic University Environmental Initiative Committee, with the leadership of then Vice President and Provost Leonard Berry, and President Anthony Catanese, provided support for the conference foundational to this work. Barbara Gray and Stanley Andrews, from the Division of Sponsored Research, Florida Atlantic University (FAU), wrote the grant leading to funding of the Environmental Initiative by Donnell–Kay Foundation.

Special thanks go to the Conference Planning Committee for the Conference on Expressions of Caring in Nursing: Exploring Our Environmental Connections, held in March 1993: Cathy Appleton, Anita Beckerman, Dean Anne Boykin, Nancie Bruce, Shirley Chesley, Sherrilyn Coffman, Diane Cope, Susan Folden, James Forrest, Nino Locsin, Mary Lucas, Patricia Munhall, Marilyn Parker, Robin Petit, Suzanne Sheber, Patricia Siccardi, Judith Stoeckman, Ceta Storms, Cathie Wallace, and Marguerite Warner.

Allan Graubard, Editorial Director, the National League for Nursing Press, provided patient, thoughtful support and guidance for which we are extremely grateful. Due to his investigation and support, NLN chose to produce this volume in an environmentally sensitive manner. Friends (both human two-footed and furry four-footed), family, and co-workers nurtured our personal energy systems as we engaged in this work. Dean Anne Boykin of FAU College of Nursing, Dean Judith Balcerski, and Associate Dean Patricia Munhall of Barry University School of Nursing gave their wholehearted support.

The efforts of all these persons, and others whom we may have left unnamed, helped to bring this book to life.

Most importantly, we are grateful to the planet and cosmos for sustaining us in our efforts. May we return, with joy, what we have been given.

Contents

Part III Extending the Domain of Nursing Knowledge through Experiencing

Part IV Nursing's Accountability to the Future

Preface

Ideas for this book began with nursing's first conference on nursing and the environment. Although the grounding for the book was the conference, contributors' most current thinking, enriched by further reflection and study, is presented here.

We believe this to be the first of many contributions whereby nurses recognize and responds specifically to who we are as humans and to how we are to live on this earth as responsible, accountable, and loving planetary citizens. Nursing will always continue to care for and be with those in need. There is growing awareness, however, that those in need include lives and forms not of the human species. Our earth is troubled in basic respects—air, soil, water, energy—and experiences systematic exploitation of animal and other life forms. Pollution and various exposures are brought about by human action and, in turn, are sources of major illnesses among humankind and beyond. Why is this happening? How might it be changed? What are root causes, beyond the symptoms we tend to treat? What is the nature of personal and professional accountability to the environment? How relevant to nursing is the emerging discipline of "environmental ethics"? Have we, as professionals, the right and responsibility to demand that our workplaces become environmentally accountable? Do we, as professionals, have the right to healthy environments in which to do healing work? What is our role, individually, in response to such questions?

This book begins to name and to address the issues and does so from a metaparadigm perspective as well as from the particulars of day-to-day practice. Contributors present and underscore a common thread running throughout the book: the issue of *the nature of our relationships*—with self, with one another, with the earth, and with all the other inhabitants of our planet. *Do* we walk in balance and in beauty and *will* we leave this home a little better than we found it?

We, as editors and authors, respectfully request that you journey with us through these pages, asking, as we have: What does all this mean to *me?* How does this inform my practice and my profession? How may I become a part of a conscious and joyous going forth?

ELEANOR A. SCHUSTER
CAROLYN L. BROWN

Boca Raton, Florida
October 1994

Foreword

It is a special privilege to introduce this path-breaking volume. A paradigm shift, toward an expanded awareness of the environment and of prevention, is clearly under way in the entire field of health care. Nurses are in the forefront of rethinking the relationships: between the human family and all the other life forms of the biosphere; between nurses and those they care for. Nurses are reweaving the roles of communities, public health education, families, and individuals, and showing them how to share the responsibilities for healthier life-styles, healthier cities, healthier economies, and healthier societies. This book fills a vast need—to reinvent our current hierarchical, bureaucratic medical–industrial complex, which is geared to high-tech crisis interventions, and emerge with a more decentralized, humanity-scaled, affordable system based on partnerships, wellness, and overall quality of life.

Let us view the current U.S. health care debate from a global, multicultural perspective. Health is a universally desirable goal. In most societies, it is linked with the goals of human development, social well-being, basic needs satisfaction, meaningful work, and aspirations for "progress" and "quality of life." All these goals cross cultures and embody visions for the future: scenarios of preferable outcomes and desirable societies. For the past 300 years, an increasing number of human societies have adopted the vision of the industrial revolution—to create a cornucopia of material goods. This vision of progress via industrialization, mass production, technological efficiency, and ever-widening mass consumption gradually became dominant. It is now time to re-assess this often beneficial social and technological revolution, reviewing environmental costs and sustainability over the long term.

Within the ideological framework of industrial progress, the human body too became viewed as a machine with identifiable and, later, replaceable parts. The growing specialization of industrial production and division of labor provided the context for later medical specialization. Academic disciplines became increasingly fragmented. The underlying Cartesian assumptions that wholes could be understood by examining their parts went largely unchallenged until anomalies piled up at the interfaces between disciplines. Eventually, they led to paradigm shifts, as described by Kuhn (1962) in *The Structure of Scientific Revolutions.* Recently, a post-Cartesian scientific paradigm has emerged that is less mechanistic and more organic and systemic. Its principles include: (1) *interconnectedness* at every system level; (2) *redistribution* and the recycling of all elements and structures; (3) *heterarchy,* intercommunication among networks, mutual causality, and self-organization; (4) *complementarity* beyond either/or dichotomous logics and zero sum games; (5) *uncertainty* from static, mechanistic, equilibrium models to living systems; and (6) *change* as fundamental.

The current health care debate is characteristic of such a paradigm shift. The extent of specialization and fragmentation has reached classic proportions: the goal of health itself is obscured by the debate about means, money, and institutional rivalries among providers. For example, a recent glossary by Slee and Slee (1994), runs to 149 pages of mind-numbing acronyms and new phrases. Meanwhile, economics has emerged as the predominant social "science"—bestriding public-sector policy making and private-sector market interactions, and claiming to incorporate models of human behavior and psychology. The crowning achievement of generations of economists was the consolidation of all industrial sectors into an overall picture: a system of national accounts (SNA). This led to the gross national product (GNP), which emerged in the United Kingdom and the United States at the onset of World War II, for the purpose of maximizing war production.

The GNP was and is an expression of the industrial paradigm: it is the measure of a society's overall production of goods and, increasingly, services, transacted in money terms. About half of all production of goods and services in industrial societies is unpaid; GNP simply ignores this portion. This cooperative "love economy," which I have described in *Paradigms in Progress* (1991), includes do-it-yourself construction and repair; growing food; caring for the sick, old, and young; volunteering in the community; serving on school boards; and maintaining households and gardens. These activities are crucially related to health outcomes and healthy communities. In developing countries, this unpaid, "informal" economy is often larger than the official GNP-measured sector, sometimes accounting for as much as 75% of all production in societies where traditional agriculture and community life are still not primarily based on money. Economics textbooks still hold that "rational" behavior is competitive maximization of self-interest; therefore, such caring, sharing, cooperative behavior is, per se, *irrational.* GNP (and its narrower version, gross domestic product, or GDP) also sets at zero the value of education, health, the environment, and the social infrastructure. The World Bank at last acknowledged, in its *World Development Report, 1993,* that development theories should not continue to overlook the unpaid cooperative production sectors, and that public health at the grass roots level should become a focus of development policies (which would also cut costs dramatically).

Yet the model of "progress as GNP growth" still holds sway in the minds of politicians and policy makers—a classic case of confusing means with ends. The goal has always been human development, but it became equated with GNP growth as the means. The anomalies that have built up over the decades since World War II include social anomalies (effects of profit maximizing in the private sector and the impact of government macroeconomic errors): jobless economic growth, increase in part-time work (contingency workers are now 30% of the U.S. work force), shuttered main streets and shattered communities, poverty gaps, violence, crime, drugs, lagging literacy rates, latch-key and street children, rising urban infant mortality, and teen pregnancies. Environmental anomalies include: pollution of air and water, and depletion of natural resources (all "free" in GNP and in economics textbooks until recently). The paradigm of progress-as-GNP-growth equated "wealth" with rising money income per capita and rising productivity per capita—an illustration of the statistical dangers of averaging. Macroeconomic policies based on such statistical illusions are akin to a doctor making her rounds in a ward containing patients with various different ailments and prescribing adrenaline for everyone. Heroically aggregated statistics like GNP obscure daily realities in peoples' lives and communities and lead to bureaucratic centralization countries and corporations. For example, GNP-measured per-capita incomes can rise when a country creates a few more millionaires, even though most of its people are poorer, as is often the case. Similarly, focusing on increasing labor productivity per capita obscures the flip side of this formula: more capital, more energy and resource intensity, more automation *and,* simultaneously, rising joblessness and welfare rolls. A more systemic focus would target energy productivity, management productivity, investment productivity, and ecological productivity.

As nurses and other health professionals know, health has more to do with socioeconomic status and job security than with the medical system. Thus, the progress-as-GNP-growth paradigm now impedes the debate about health care. The debate ranges from *Business Week's* editorial of May 2, 1994, stating that the health crisis is "mostly an insurance problem," to the view of the past president of the American Medical Association, Edward R. Annis (1993), that the system is "on the verge of collapse." Today's medical systems and their iatrogenic casualties now account for more than 100,000 deaths and over 1 million injuries by medical malpractice in U.S. hospitals, according to Wachsman and Alschuler (1993). GNP-driven economic growth also produces human pathologies. If GNP growth remains the centerpiece of public policy, then the burgeoning medical industries ameliorating GNP's social and environmental costs (morbidity and mortality due to stress, auto accidents, guns and violent crimes, substance abuse, sedentary life-styles, workplace and environmental toxicity) will continue growing. All these social costs are still *added into* GNP (instead of subtracted from), as if they were more production and a good thing. Every time there is an auto accident or an oil spill, the GNP goes up. Life-style changes toward healthier habits, less consumption, more walking, and so on, *decrease* GNP. Nurses have known all this for a long time, because they are close to patients and because they, unlike doctors today, so often deliver care in home settings.

Today's perverse economics cannot account for long-term outcomes or prevention. As I pointed out earlier (Henderson, 1981), a vast, shadowy, social-costs-based "mirror image" of GNP was clearly identifiable. This undifferentiated national accounting system included such costs as the stress industry (then some $70 billion annually); the environmental cleanup and pollution control industry; the psychiatric and community counseling industry (to assist the poor and underemployed); the bottled water industry; and others. Today, we can add the punishment industry (purveyors of electronic restraining bracelets, prison builders, and so on); the private security industry (guards, locks, mace, alarm systems, pilferage prevention, weapons). We cannot even clarify which are costs and which are benefits because the system is circular and interactive, not linear as described in economics textbooks. Every category of social cost and amelioration of GNP-growth's effects has now spawned its own "parasitic" industry, trade association, lobbyists, and ranks of employees. For example, the $1 trillion medical industry now provides one in ten of all U.S. jobs. Tobacco companies, recently under renewed congressional attack, herded their employees to Washington to lobby for protection of their jobs. As the voices in this book show so clearly, nurses are in the forefront of reinventing such irrational bureaucracies by expanding the scope of their analyses to embrace broader social and environmental contexts. Complex societies can be effectively governed and restructured to be more user-friendly by using feedback from individual voters and consumers using dynamic, interactive, systems models. These models and policies must be interdisciplinary; they might include new quality-of-life indicators; technology assessments; environmental and social impact analyses; risk assessment; game theory; and chaos models.

Feedback from individuals in more decentralized communities and enterprises can be linked laterally, via increased communications networks, to make societies more manageable. As organizational theorists Warren Bennis and Philip Slater pointed out in 1964, democracies have become necessary: feedback in the form of votes is essential for decision makers in complex institutions. Another vital form of feedback from individuals is the price system. But if they are to guide producers, prices must accurately reflect all the true social and environmental costs of production. Needless to say, in a market-dominated society, few economists are hired to quantify these broader costs—the "bads" that come along with the goods; the disservices and disamenities passed along to taxpayers and future generations. Other important feedbacks to decision makers include mass media, citizen organizations, regulations, lawsuits and tort liabilities, and books like this one, as well as all the longer feedback loops from Mother Nature: the earth's thinning ozone layer, dying forests, increasing desertification, and lost biodiversity. Emerging viruses set loose by ecosystem disturbances such as logging and clear-cutting forests are another "early warning" feedback to human policies, as Morse (1993) has pointed out. Many such feedback loops are brought to the attention of decision makers and voters by the use of new quality-of-life indicators to flesh out their "instrument panels."

As we are learning, industrial societies focused on the GNP-growth formula are simply unsustainable, because they cannibalize their own resources and eventually exploit their own people. After a certain level of industrialization is reached, societies become addicted to increased government spending at all levels (to coordinate all the complexity) and to consumerism. Such averaged levels of consumption (in the United States, consumerism accounts for 65% of GNP) must be hyped by credit and advertising geared to frivolous, trivial desires, sometimes fostering addictions, for example, abuse of over-the-counter drugs, junk foods, and so on. By the same token, the poor often go without necessities while succumbing to TV-promoted, socially induced, harmful patterns of consumption. Further, pollution of our air, water, food, and land in pursuit of GNP-measured growth accelerates morbidity and weakening of human immunity.

This is why I honor the work of the authors of this book, as well as other innovators such as Dr. Ilona Kickbusch, the World Health

Organization (WHO), and all those pioneers of the Healthy Cities movement who are redefining health, wealth, and progress from the grass roots upward. The Quality Indicators for Progress, used in Jacksonville, Florida, and pioneered by Dr. Marion Chambers, have tracked community health since 1983. The obvious way to break out of this GNP-growth trap is to account on a current basis for all these social and environmental costs, sooner or later passed on to taxpayers, and get them back onto the balance sheets of producing companies so that they show up in the correct, full-cost pricing of all products. Further, the new quality-of-life indicators, which use statistics from many disciplines, can serve to target healthier community goals and provide early warning of problems we may otherwise continue to sweep under the rug, pass on to future generations, or address via inflationary deficit-spending. All this is common sense when wider environmental analyses are used, such as those in this volume.

Mass production economies first needed advertising and credit to fuel mass consumption. The current economic U.S. recovery was largely fueled by an increase in consumer debt; the ratio to disposable income rose to 16.5% in January 1994, and is still rising. Industrial economies have become addicted to ever more waste of energy and raw materials. Today, they are also addicted to spurious product differentiation and technological innovation and ever larger doses of capital investment as they chase their own tails. In today's globalization of technology, finance, information, work, and migration, every country will end up losing in the mad competition for production efficiency and export-led growth—auctioning off their work forces, public sector assets, cultural heritage, and environmental resources to the highest bidder in exchange for volatile paper and electronic currencies (Kurtzman, 1993). This is now spreading as Eastern European and Russian officials adopt outdated 19th-century capitalism from U.S. textbooks and the emerging Asian players—China, Indonesia, Malaysia, and Thailand—are urged to follow suit.

In the United States, we played out the drama of the industrial paradigm to the hilt, with all its good and bad news. The 1993 Detroit Jobs Summit targeted "structural joblessness issues," including health costs, aging populations, and "inefficient" labor markets.

Such old paradigm views also seek to cut social safety-net legislation and blame fringe benefits and minimum wages, rather than automation-favoring tax credits, for pricing labor out of markets. Yet, in the United States, average total compensation (including such fringe benefits) is *lower* after inflation than in 1987. The real problem, buried in a *Business Week* (July 12, 1993) article, is the *relative* cost of labor vis-à-vis capital—exacerbated by productivity formulas and tax incentives. In a global economy, investors are free to roam worldwide rather than create domestic jobs, which will require *employment tax credits.* Together with full-cost prices for energy and virgin raw materials and value extracted taxes (VET) to discourage waste and pollution, all economies can run on a leaner mix of capital, energy, and materials, and a richer mix of human resources. Such basic shifts can redirect economies toward fuller employment—even if the new jobs perforce will be in a restructured medical sector. For example, restructuring of U.S. medicine is already evidenced by the 425 million visits Americans made in 1990 to nonconventional practitioners (acupuncturists; holistic, naturopathic, and biofeedback specialists, and so on)—about 10% more than the 388 million visits logged by all U.S. primary care physicians (Eisenberg, 1993). Pollution control, environmental cleanup, and a more people-intensive, decentralized health care sector, together with developing more efficient, "greener" technologies, companies, and public services, will provide millions of jobs in the late 1990s. Introducing employment tax credits and VET, particularly for small companies and the self-employed, can help. For example, such assistance to the unemployed and self-employed in Britain has raised self-employment to 11% of the work force as well as creating 650,000 new small businesses. Many nurses may find that independent professional, group, and alternative settings, such as birthing centers, home birthing, and delivery of other health services, are more efficient and congenial for them and those in their care.

The wholesale redefining of health, wealth, and progress, as WHO has also found, is a worldwide phenomenon. As opinion research by DYG, Inc., for the Healthcare Forum, shows, in maturing industrial societies, like the United States, people are again focusing on the fundamentals. They include the need to redefine goals and values, buttress the family, and work cooperatively to achieve healthier communities and quality of life. This new focus may at last lead to proper accounting of the unpaid goods and services of the love economy, as a less-costly alternative to higher taxes for more government-provided social services. At the United Nations Earth Summit in Rio de Janeiro in 1992, citizens' organizations from over 170 countries gathered to share such new definitions and press new paradigms of progress and development onto their government representatives. They drafted treaties to protect children, women, small farmers, neighborhoods, families, communities, and the rights of indigenous peoples, and to preserve cultural diversity as well as biodiversity. They focused on the *causes* of poverty and jobless economic growth generated by the faulty GNP formula. Many produced charters and principles for an emerging Earth Ethics that acknowledged humans as one species within the web of all life on this planet. They redefined the concept of security beyond military terms—civil and job security, environmental security—as a security of individuals rather than the state. These citizens represented a "third force" arising in the world: a global civil society to check, balance, and augment the capacities of today's two major planetary institutions: nation states and global corporations. Citizens and their voluntary organizations (which the United Nations insists on calling "non-governmental organizations"—NGOs) are a major source of social innovation in all countries, as I have described elsewhere (Henderson, 1993).

Today, social innovation is becoming ever more vital as global change speeds up and continues restructuring all societies. This book is a prime example of such social innovation. The citizens' groups at the Rio Summit, whether their focus was human rights, poverty, worker safety, urban or rural issues, or environmental protection, urged their governments to overhaul their systems of national accounts. They drew attention to the many ways that GNP scorecards had driven countries' policies off course. The Agenda 21 agreements signed at Rio by 178 governments called for reformulating GNP to account for environmental assets and productivity, and costs of pollution and depletion, and including unpaid production and informal sectors. In February 1994, after a decade of back-room debate between traditional macroeconomists and a handful of social and statistical innovators, a new *System of National Accounts, 1993* (SNA) was published, representing joint agreements on new statistical protocols by the International Monetary Fund (IMF), the World Bank, the Organization for Economic Cooperation and Development (OECD), the European Union, and the United Nations Statistical Division.

This new international SNA will lead to new GNP formulas that are more systemic, but by no means perfect. At least, new SNAs will address the need to account for infrastructure and environmental resources as a country's capital assets. In April 1994, the U.S. Bureau of Economic Analysis, which had been busy recalculating GNP for the past year, announced the methods it will use to account for such environmental assets and losses due to pollution and depletion. The new "Green GNP" is not very much better and has been criticized by environmental groups. At least, we will no longer run our country as a business in a liquidation sale but will have a "net worth" statement that will, hopefully, better differentiate investments in productive capital assets (such as infrastructure, health, and education) from spending items in the national budget. Little progress is yet evident in any country on properly valuing the unpaid, cooperative production in the love economy, which is so crucial to health. Other major intangible assets of all countries are not yet carried on the books. These include: healthy, well-educated, responsible citizens; high literacy rates; good prenatal care; low infant mortality and crime rates; stable, demographically balanced populations; and personal security in safe, healthy communities. Thus, the Healthy Cities movement is more vital than ever, and those cities and communities that already use quality-of-life indicators can serve as models to teach macroeconomists how to expand and further overhaul national accounts. Nurses such as those represented in this volume are exerting their own leadership in this great paradigms shift.

To this end, my own Country Futures Indicators (CFI)© has been, for the last five years, offered as an alternative scorecard to assist societies in developing more sustainably, using a healthier recipe and valuing all the ingredients of their total productive capacity. The first working model of CFI is now being prepared for the United States in cooperation with the Calvert Group, Inc. of

Washington, DC, and its family of socially responsible investment funds, as the *Calvert-Henderson Quality-of-Life Indicators.* The CFI is unbundled and interdisciplinary; it uses the best statistics from many sectors, sources, and perspectives. CFI is, therefore, transparent to the public, allowing citizens to follow those aspects of quality of life that are of most concern to them, so that they can hold politicians accountable. Such unbundled indicators of all major aspects of quality of life allow citizens and voters to express *their own* values. This is in contrast to the macroeconomic formulas such as GDP, which permit economists to "weight," in money coefficients, all those different aspects and make their own value judgments as to whether, for example, clean air is more important than improved literacy or more money incomes. These methods are now revealed as value-laden and unscientific; worse, they preempt the very heart of the participatory, democratic feedback process.

The health care debate, to which this book contributes so splendidly, can proceed within the newly expanded paradigm of quality of life, including community health and individual responsibility for wellness, and incorporating a vision of truly human development that is ecologically sustainable. Conservatives are correct in pointing out that we can no longer just throw more money at our perverse, wasteful medical sector. Bill Clinton, when he was the Democratic candidate, was also right in campaigning for reform that would claim the some $200 billion annual savings identified in 1989 by *Consumer Reports.* The entire apparatus of the medical sector does, indeed, need restructuring and downsizing, as do so many other wasteful, unsustainable sectors that now render our economy obsolete and uncompetitive. This needed restructuring is unlikely to happen without the ongoing, gigantic war between the medical special interests being waged in the U.S. Congress. Such special interests in the status quo have already "invested" some $75 million in Congressional candidates in the past decade, according to Common Cause.

Refocusing on goals of *health,* and healthier life-styles and communities, requires education and revaluing of simple satisfactions, as this book points out. Warm relationships, families, and neighbors; meaningful work in communities where volunteering is honored; and clean air, water, and natural environments *are* more valuable than new cars, video games, fashions, or even high-tech medical "miracles." Medical hype continues to feed fantasies that, in turn, feed insatiable demands for more medical services. As in other sectors, technological innovation in the medical sector is driven by the capital investment subsidies in the tax code, mentioned earlier. The U.S. Office of Technology Assessment should continue assessing the factors that drive medical care toward excessive high-tech approaches. All this is similarly reflected in the debate over what we mean by "wealth" and "progress" nationally and internationally. The new SNAs and the complementary scorecards of progress and quality of life at the city and national levels can help people and communities to ask the right questions and focus on their long-term goals and deepest values.

Values actually drive all economic and technological systems. If they are life-affirming, systemic, long-term, and ecologically aware, such value systems (i.e., "software") are *resources* just like coal, oil, and biodiversity. Value systems are packages of software that serve the crucial function of helping human populations fit their environmental niches and adapt to changing conditions. What economics textbooks call an "economy" is simply a set of rules based on different cultural DNA codes, as I have described earlier (Henderson, 1981, 1988). These cultural DNA codes—the values, goals, and traditions of different societies—actually determine "economic" outcomes. In fact, game theory is often a more appropriate tool to study such human behavior and rules of interaction. All economies today are mixtures of markets and regulations about which today's economists have no theories. Economists would need to defer to cultural anthropologists in understanding the differing development patterns of, for example, Sweden, Taiwan, Germany, Japan, China, or Russia. This understanding of the many cultural faces of capitalism has reintroduced creativity into sterile thinking and debates left over from the Cold War. There is widely shared understanding that social safety nets, which have evolved over the past years, are necessary, in every society, to tame markets.

Today's information revolution can foster the growing global civil society, not only through today's "narrow casting" on expensive E-mail systems on Internet, but also by expanding their broadcasting capabilities and by linking their television facilities and producers. An incipient Global Television Consortium for Sustainable Development can redress today's global TV monoculture with fresh multicultural programming and news of grass-roots solutions and innovations. Television and computers are already linking patients and doctors for remote care in many countries. There will be less need to leave the beauty of natural, unspoiled habitations and the satisfactions of traditional culture for job searches in polluted, crime-infested, urban areas. Every village can have access to opportunities, education, health care, new technologies, and a rich variety of cultural contacts, as well as global, regional, and local news. The currently dominant commercial television, driven by tax-deductible advertising of unsustainable consumption and wasteful energy-intensive life-styles, will also need to be taxed. Forms of advertising that use psychological manipulation and undercut self-esteem will need to be curbed, along with excessive violence, in spite of protestations from U.S. movie and video makers that this would infringe First Amendment rights of free speech. It is already generally accepted that "free speech" does not include the right to advertise heroin, cocaine, or tobacco over the public air waves.

Implementing health care reform does not require enormous new sums of money, but it needs shifting priorities, taxes, and national budgets. Similarly, the Agenda 21 global environmental agreements, signed in 1992 at Rio, can largely be implemented if countries merely stop financing *un*sustainability. In both cases, it will then be necessary for countries to comb through their policies and priorities and muster support to remove perverse subsidies, waste, and counterproductive taxation. The growing world court of public opinion can help in refocusing from military concepts of security to human security for people rather than governments. New civilian and infrastructure investments of the growing global peace dividends will provide new jobs in sustainable development, domestically and internationally, as described in the United Nations' *Human Development Report, 1994.*

A society that has developed and maintains a resourceful value system can remain a flexible, open, learning society capable of evolving new paradigms appropriate to map and cope with emerging conditions. As the United Nations approaches its 50th anniversary, the Social Summit to be held in Copenhagen, Denmark, in March 1995, will take up all of the issues short-changed in the drive for industrial progress and GNP growth. As the new formula—sustainable human development—gradually replaces GNP growth, a large "prevention dividend" (of avoided costs) can become available as we shift from expensive, crises-driven, technological-fix, national policies. Having to keep cleaning up messes (from orbiting space debris to nuclear wastes) while we continue to replace functioning communities with dysfunctional markets is massively costly. Like the peace dividend—which has accrued since 1989, thanks to a 3% average decline in world military spending amounting to $935 billion—the "prevention dividend" will be vast as we redirect our GNP toward the new priorities of sustainable development measured by quality-of-life indicators and geared to longer-term goals.

Such new policies to unleash virtuous circles can target longer-term efficiency and healthier communities. Our definition of "prevention" will need to be precise: as *software,* that is, value shifts, social learning, life-style changes, and better policies and indicators. Prevention in this societal sense is needed much more than preventive, diagnostic medical hardware, which, quite rightly, is often deemed excessively expensive. The real payoff will be in a shift back to values of family, community, and nature, and a shift forward to early-warning research scenarios, and longer-term concerns beyond those of individual textbook economics self-interest. Indeed, the caring and medical professions have been distorted by this self-interest economic model. Rodwin (1993) describes seven physicians' conflicts of interest: (1) kickbacks to and from medical suppliers; (2) physicians' self-referral to facilities in which they invest; (3) physicians' selling of medical products; (4) hospital purchase of physicians' practices; (5) payments made by hospitals to recruit physicians; (6) gift from medical suppliers; (7) physicians' risk-sharing in HMOs and hospitals. Codes of medical ethics ignore these conflicts of interest. Corporations are internalizing many formerly externalized social and environmental costs because of insurance liability, consumer and public pressure, better information, and socially responsible, patient investors. The Calvert Social

Investment Funds have amply demonstrated the breadth of this new market of concerned, long-term investors, now approaching $700 billion and spreading worldwide.

Several authors in this book refer to the original Native American inhabitants of this continent. They used the concept of evaluating policies for their future effects, at least on the Seventh Generation hence. Markets, like technology, can be used appropriately, but both are bad masters. There are at least five levels of policy interventions, social innovations, and new market opportunities if we are to make our global economy sustainable for the Seventh Generation and beyond:

1. *Individuals and families* can become more responsible for their own wellness and life-styles; balance consumerism with more nonmaterial satisfactions; personal development, relationships, and community. They can recycle and reuse, or buy environmentally friendly products from socially responsible companies and local merchants; invest in such companies as well as in local credit unions. They can form buying clubs with other families and contract with local farms for clean, organically grown produce. They can form skills exchange networks and cocounseling and service credit programs, and participate in local volunteering and policy making at all levels.

2. *Communities and local governments* can change zoning to accommodate closer living and working patterns, home-based business, and intentional families; enact policies for recycling, energy efficiency, solar retrofits, bike lanes, pedestrian paths, and "traffic calming"; and set up service credit and local exchange systems. For example, a Miami architectural firm, Duany and Plater-Zyberk, estimate that such rezoning could save an average family $5,000 annually in transportation costs.

3. *Corporations* can offer employees wellness programs, fitness training, and incentives such as day care, car pooling, and flex time. They can redesign their products to reduce social and environmental impacts while internalizing all costs into prices. Annual reports should contain state-of-the-art, social, and environmental audits. They can initiate team-based total

quality management and other innovative human resource management programs, and thereby flatten hierarchies.

4. *National governments* can stop subsidizing unsustainability (e.g., oil depletion allowances) and ill health (e.g., subsidies to tobacco growers), and shift tax codes toward rewarding healthy life-styles, productive employment, and investments in new companies offering environmentally advanced technologies and socially innovative services. Sin taxes should include pollution, waste, planned obsolescence, and resource depletion. Governments can continue overhauling systems of national accounts, expand GNP, and publish interdisciplinary quality-of-life indicators, as described.

5. *International* playing fields must now be leveled *upward,* not downward, by negotiating treaties and agreements to raise the global base level. National governments need to *recognize* those policy areas where they have lost control to global forces (global corporations and markets), so as to begin scheduling negotiations among all those countries affected. Some of the girder work under this more ethical floor is already in place with global agreements on health, worker safety, consumer and environmental protection, and the agreements signed on ozone depletion and biodiversity. As other provisions of Agenda 21 and other reforms are implemented, it should be possible to change today's global economic warfare into a "win-win" world game where the most ethical countries and companies can win.

As this book amply demonstrates, healthy environments, healthy societies, and healthy economies are all essential preconditions for healthy communities and people. Today's creative challenges can provide productive employment for everyone willing and able to work. In longer time horizons, all our self-interests are identical and the new Earth Ethics is simply becoming pragmatic.

HAZEL HENDERSON

St. Augustine, Florida
August 1994

ABOUT THE AUTHOR

Hazel Henderson is an independent futurist, syndicated columnist, and consultant on sustainable development in over 30 countries. Her editorial columns are syndicated by Inter Press Service worldwide and by the Los Angeles Times-Mirror Syndicate. She has published articles in over 250 journals. Her most recent book is *Paradigms In Progress* (1991). The first version of her Country Futures Indicators (CFI)© (an alternative to Gross National Product, GNP) will be launched as a co-venture with the Calvert Group, Inc., as the Calvert-Henderson Quality-of-Life Indicators in early 1995.

She serves on many boards, including the Calvert Social Investment Fund, the Cousteau Society, the Council on Economic Priorities, the Worldwatch Institute, and on editorial boards including *World Paper, Futures Research Quarterly, Futures,* and the *Journal of Inter-Disciplinary Economics* (U.K.). She serves on the Business Council on Sustainable Development Task Force on Eco-Efficiency in Global Capital Markets (Geneva), is a Fellow of the World Business Academy, and a member of the Business Council for the World Summit on Social Development of the UN (Paris). Henderson also serves on the new Global Commission to Fund the United Nations and is co-guest editor (with Harlan Cleveland) of the special issue of *Futures: The UN at 50: Policy and Financing Alternatives* (Elsevier Scientific Pub. Co., March, 1995). She was a discussant at the UN Roundtable on Global Change in Stockholm, July, 1994. She has been Regent's Lecturer at the University of California (Santa Barbara) and held the Horace Albright Chair in Conservation at the University of California (Berkeley), and served on the U.S. Congress Office of Technology Assessment Advisory Council from 1974–1980. She is a Limited Partner of the Global Environment Fund (Washington, D.C.), a member of the Social Venture Network, and a Limited Partner and advisor to the Sino-American Development Corporation (New York, NY).

REFERENCES

Annis, E. R. (1993). *Code blue: Health care in crisis.* American Medical Association.

Bennis, W., & Slater, P. Editorial, *Harvard Business Review,* 1964.

DYG, Inc. *Healthcare Forum.* (Title unavailable)

Consumer Reports, 1989. (Title unavailable)

Business Week, July 12, 1993. (Title unavailable)

Business Week, May 2, 1994. (Title unavailable)

Eisenberg, D. *New England Journal of Medicine,* January 28, 1993. (Title unavailable)

Henderson, H. (1981). *Politics of the solar age.* Indianapolis, IN: Knowledge Systems.

Henderson, H. (1991). *Paradigms in progress.* Indianapolis, IN: Knowledge Systems.

Henderson, H. (1993). Social innovations and citizen movements.

Futures, pp. 322–338, Vol. 25, #3 (April, 1993).

International Monetary Fund (IMF), World Bank, OECD, European Nation, & United Nations Statistical Division. (February 1994). *System of National Accounts, 1993.*

Kuhn, T. (1962). *The structure of scientific revolutions.*

Kurtzman, J. (1993). *The death of money: How the electronic economy has destabilized the world's markets and created financial chaos.* New York: Simon & Schuster.

Morse, S. S. (1993). *Emerging viruses.* New York: Oxford University Press.

Rodwin, M. A. (1993). *Medicine, money and morals.* New York: Oxford University Press.

Slee, V. N., & Slee, D. A. (1994). *Health care reform terms.* 2nd ed. St. Paul, MN: Tringa Press.

United Nations. (1994). *Human Development Report, 1994.* Washington, D.C.: U.S. Government Printing Office.

U.S. Bureau of Economic Analysis. (April 1994). *Calculations of 1993 GNP.* Washington, D.C.: U.S. Government Printing Office.

Wachsman, H. F., & Alschuler, S. (1993). *Lethal medicine.* New York: Henry Holt.

World Bank. World Development Report, 1993. Washington, D.C.: U.S. Government Printing Office.

PART

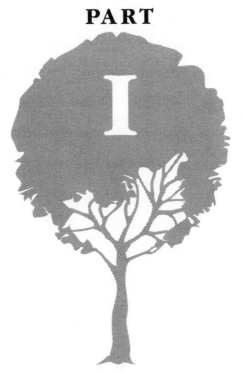

Environment as a Domain of Nursing Knowledge

The phrase *domain of nursing knowledge* calls forth old images of ownership, territoriality, and control. We use the word *domain* in the sense of laying claim to an area of knowledge development for nursing. Chapters in this part provide readers with an expanded vision of what nursing is now, and what it can be as we move into the future. All of us are shaped by and contribute to shaping the environments that form the context for our lives. As you explore these chapters, we invite you to allow yourself to see both the rich history and the potential of nurses' place in creating a sustainable future.

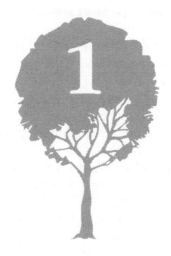

The Environment: Alive, Whole, and Interacting

Dorothy Kleffel*

Nurses care for the casualties of adverse environmental situations, but are strangely silent about directly addressing environmental contributors to poor health. For instance, a nurse may give compassionate care to a child who has leukemia, but seldom will she or he get involved with ensuring the cleanup of a toxic dump located near the child's home. Pollution of all kinds, homelessness, hazards in the workplace, and the ravages of war are examples of destructive environmental conditions that we hear about or experience every day. These environmental influences affect the health and well-being of humans and all other living things.

*The author acknowledges the American Nurses Foundation for partial financial support for the research on which this chapter is based.

The issue of nurses' not becoming involved with broad environmental concerns had long puzzled me. I was active in the environmental movement and knew that poor environmental conditions were precursors to poor health. Because the health of people is a concern of nurses, it seemed reasonable to me that nurses would be interested in addressing environmental concerns in order to enhance the well-being of humans.

These ideas led me to focus on many aspects of the environment during my doctoral studies, and to view the environment as a major concept of nursing knowledge for my dissertation. In this chapter, I describe the background of the research and some the study's more salient findings.

ENVIRONMENT AS A MAJOR CONCEPT OF NURSING

The environment has been a major concept in the realm of nursing knowledge since the time of Florence Nightingale, who was a part of the great sanitarian reform movement of her day. Emphasizing the importance of creating an optimal environment so that healing could take place, Nightingale believed that nursing actions should continue to be focused thereon (Nightingale, 1969/1860).

Notwithstanding Nightingale's emphasis, how do modern nursing scholars understand the environment? Reviewing major nurse theorists' ideas about the environment, I found, as had Chopoorian in 1986, that they generally regarded the environment as the individual's immediate surroundings or circumstances, to be managed or controlled or to which the individual must adapt or conform (Kleffel, 1991). They did not address broad dimensions of the environment such as the social, economic, and political aspects that can be either precursors to illnesses or enhancers of well-being. I agreed with Meleis (1991), who wrote that modern nursing scholars still regard the environment as a major construct of nursing science but have not addressed it with the same depth and conviction as did Nightingale.

Nor have nurse researchers addressed broad environmental concerns. I did a manual literature search to try to locate nursing research within these larger environmental realms. I searched from the year 1961 to February 1991 (Kleffel, 1991), and later updated the search to 1994 (Kleffel, 1994) and found only one nursing research on the broad environmental influences of health. I concluded that, although nurses care for persons whose conditions are connected with environmental degradation, they have not addressed the larger physical, social, cultural, political, and economic elements relating to the health and welfare of people. As I progressed through the doctoral program, I began to think about how I could incorporate these ideas into my dissertation.

THE STUDY

During my reading, I identified several nursing scholars from the literature who, rather than regarding the environment as the immediate surroundings or situations of the person, had addressed larger environmental concerns. They focused on addressing the broad physical, social, cultural, political, economic, and global factors that are related to health. I decided that I wanted to interview them to see how they perceived an ideal environmental domain of nursing, and what action they believed nurses should take in relation to the environment.

I used combined qualitative research methods for data collection and analysis. I conducted four initial interviews using qualitative approaches (Strauss & Corbin, 1991) that incorporated feminist values of nonhierarchy, subjectivity, contexuality, reciprocity, and empowerment (Anderson, 1991). Then I conducted a focus group of nine participants. The strength of using a focus group in addition to individual interviews is the opportunity to collect data from group interaction (Morgan, 1988). The data from the individual interviews and the focus group were further enriched by four additional interviews. I analyzed the data by using the constant comparative method, which consists of concurrent data collection and analysis (Strauss & Corbin, 1991). This method is congruent with data analysis recommended for focus groups (Kingry, Tiedje, & Friedman, 1990). The study was informed by an ecofeminist framework, which is a synthesis of environmental and feminist theories (Warren, 1987). The question that I wanted to answer was:

What is an ideal environmental domain of nursing knowledge as envisioned by scholars who had addressed broad environmental dimensions in their work?

OUR ALIVE, WHOLE, AND INTERACTING ENVIRONMENT

In contrast to the circumscribed ideas of environment of the major nurse theorists and the work done by nurse researchers, my participants spoke of a dynamic world of unity and wholeness with numerous patterns and complexities, of which we are mostly unaware. Some of these patterns were identified as dimensions (physical, social, cultural, economic, political, space/time, ontological, and everyday life), and levels (micro, meso, macro, global, universal, and cosmological) that are alive, interconnected, and in constant interaction. The boundaries between the various patterns and complexities were considered as either open, or fluid and overlapping. The patterns of the environment are within the whole, and the whole is reflected within the patterns.

Our alive, whole, and interacting planet was considered by many of the participants as part of a universe that is also alive, whole, and interacting. Our universe, in turn, is situated on the edge of a cosmos. From the perspective of some of the participants, any activity at any level reverberates throughout the cosmos.

Conceiving of the environment as alive, whole, and interacting is currently not in the mainstream of Western scientific thought. However, these ideas have existed throughout time. I will discuss both ancient and modern philosophies that incorporate these perspectives into their worldview.

Ancient and Modern Environmental Worldviews

The idea that the earth is alive, whole, and interacting has existed since ancient Greek and Roman times, about 2000 years ago. Early

Eastern and Native American philosophies also reflect this dynamic and unitary view of the world. Modern environmental thought, such as the Gaia hypothesis, holographic theory, and deep ecology, appears to be an update of these early ideas.

The concepts of alive, whole, and interacting are, in actuality, entwined and overlapping. They are discussed separately in this section for purposes of analyses.

Alive. The view that the earth is a living organism was held by many ancient systems of thought. The world as an alive entity was personified by the Earth goddess of the ancient Greeks and Romans. Mother Earth was the oldest and greatest goddess. She bore all that there is: the sky, the stars, all worlds, and all creatures. This view of the Earth goddess later gave way to a less personalized perspective that the earth is one vast, alive, sentient organism (Hughes, 1982).

Similar views of the earth as a living organism are held by traditional Native American cultures. Although they are numerous, they share a core belief that the earth is a living, conscious being that must be treated with respect and care (Booth & Jacobs, 1990). The American Indian regarded all entities (such as the sky, clouds, wind, rocks, soil, streams, trees, insects, birds, and animals) as having consciousness and reason as complete as humans (Callicott, 1982).

Many ancient Eastern philosophies also incorporated the living characteristics of the environment into their systems of thought. For example, in Taoism, a Chinese philosophy, ch'i is the living vital force of the cosmos. The least intelligent being, such as a rock, and the highest manifestation of spirituality, such as heaven, consist of the living ch'i. Nature is the result of fusion and merging of vital forces that form the great harmony. Nothing is outside of nature (Wei-Ming, 1989).

These ideas of the world as dynamic and living, held by ancient thinkers, are reflected in contemporary environmental thought. The Gaia hypothesis (Lovelock, 1979, 1988) is considered to be an update of the ancient Greco-Roman organic notion. Gaia is a system made up of all living things and their environment. There is no clear distinction, only graded intensities, between living and nonliving matter.

Other environmental approaches include within their frameworks the concept of a living planet. Some ecofeminists, in their efforts to construct a more just and peaceful society, are reclaiming early Greek, Roman, Native American, and Eastern ideas of a living world (Eisler, 1990). Deep ecologists believe that there is no firm division within the field of existence—no boundaries between human and nonhuman realms, because all are alive (Devall & Sessions, 1985). Bohm (1980), one of the early developers of holographic theory, believed that life and intelligence are present in the fabric of the entire universe; in energy, space, and time, as well as in all matter.

Conceiving of everything as being alive may be difficult for those of us who live in the modern West. Jerome Rothstein, a physicist, used an analogy of a giant redwood tree in explaining how rocks are alive. The great redwood tree is an ancient spire of dead wood, made of lignin and cellulose produced by the predecessors of the living cells of the tree's bark. Likewise, in the earth, many of the atoms of the rocks, clear down into the magma layer of the earth, were once part of the ancestral life from which we all have come (cited in Lovelock, 1988).

Whole.   Wholeness was another theme incorporated in several ancient philosophies. The world was considered whole by the ancient Greeks and Romans, first with the concept of the Mother Earth goddess, then later as an enormous, single entity. Traditional Native Americans considered all human and natural realms as unified and akin (Callicott, 1982). In Taoism, the earth was considered an organic whole comprised of all patterns of nature. Humans are one part of the whole and must act within natural laws (Peerenboom, 1992).

The idea of wholeness is a theme in many current environmental philosophies. For instance, in the Gaia hypothesis, all of earth's matter forms a complex system of life, which is one living organism. This unitary organism has faculties and powers far beyond those of its constituent parts (Lovelock, 1979). In holographic theory, the universe is conceived as a giant hologram. Every portion of the universe is reflected within each part, and every part enfolds the whole (Bohm, 1980). In other words, every leaf or every cell in our world reflects the entire cosmos. Deep ecologists believe that all organisms and entities in the ecosphere are parts of the interrelated whole and are equal in intrinsic value (Devall & Sessions, 1985).

Interacting.   Environmental interaction was considered to be of great importance by the participants in my focus group. Some believed that nursing's focus on interaction is unique to the profession.

According to the ancient Greeks, Mother Earth interacts with and nourishes all creatures. If we serve her well, she gives us good things in return. If we treat her poorly, the balance tips, resulting in famine, disease, disaster, and death (Hughes, 1982). As the Mother Earth image gave way to a less personal but still whole and living organism, the Greeks emphasized the interactions and balance of the elements and creatures within the unity of the world. Humans are one functioning part of the totality and act in harmony within the organism. Environmental problems reflect disharmony and illness of the organism (Hughes, 1982).

Traditional Native Americans believe in the kinship of all things in a sort of universal relatedness that is part of the Great Spirit. Plants, animals, rocks, thunder clouds, and stars, for example, are all part of the traditional familylike relationships (Neihardt, 1931). Native Americans hunted and gathered in a way that preserved environmental balance. For anything that was taken, something had to be offered in return. Species did not become endangered or exterminated because the Native Americans did not want to eliminate a kindred being. Disease and calamity result if these reciprocal relationships and interactions do not take place (Booth & Jacobs, 1990).

Ancient Chinese philosophers considered Tao as nature. Tao is nameless, intangible, empty, simple, all-pervasive, eternal, life-sustaining, and nourishing. It is a process of change and interaction governed by the interactions of Ying and Yang. There is no chasm between humans and nature because everything is connected to everything else. Everything is ontologically equal; therefore, humans receive no special status or attention (Ip,

1983). To cultivate the environment is to cultivate oneself. To use the environment in an adverse manner is to impoverish oneself (Ames, 1986).

Modern environmental ideas also include themes of interconnectedness and interrelatedness. Arne Naess (1973), a Norwegian philosopher who developed the principles of deep ecology, viewed the environment as a relational total field. He rejected the person-in-the-environment image in favor of one where all organisms are "knots in the biospherical net" (p. 95). He considered all organisms and entities as parts of the interrelated whole; if we harm the rest of nature, then we harm ourselves. Everything is interrelated, and there are no boundaries (Duvall & Sessions, 1985).

In the Gaia hypothesis, Lovelock (1988) described all ecosystems as being connected. To represent the interconnections, he used the analogy of an animal's liver, which has some capacity to regulate its internal environment. Although cells of the liver can be grown in isolation, neither the animal without its liver, nor the liver itself, can live independently. Both depend on the interconnections they share. Gaia, as a totality involving the Earth's biosphere, atmosphere, oceans, and soil, constitutes a feedback system that seeks an optimal environment for life on this planet. An unbalanced environment, caused either by natural events or by humans, can have disastrous consequences for life (Lovelock, 1979).

In holographic theory, interactions begin at the atomic level. Bohm (1980) found that when electrons and ions were in plasma, they stopped behaving like individuals and began behaving as if they were a part of a larger interconnected whole. He believed that everything in the universe is part of a continuum. Although things appear separate, everything is a seamless extension of and ultimately blends into everything else. Ignoring of this dynamic interconnectedness of all things is responsible for many of our problems. For instance, we believe that we can extract valuable parts of the earth without affecting the whole, and we believe that it is possible to treat parts of the body and not be concerned with the whole (Talbot, 1991).

Some common ideas about the environment being alive, whole, and interacting can be identified from the above discussion. When we conceptualize an environment that is alive, we mean that everything within the planet is living. Soil, rocks, atmosphere, oceans, space/time, plants, all creatures, and so forth, make up the living structure of our planet. This organismic characteristic of our planet extends to the universe and throughout the cosmos. The living quality of our environment is unified and whole.

When we speak of the environment that is whole, we are speaking of one huge entity that is comprised of many patterns or elements that are united into a whole that is greater than its elements. This whole of our earth is a part of the whole universe, which is part of a whole cosmos.

When we speak of interacting, we mean that all of the elements and patterns that exist within the whole are interwoven, interconnected, and interrelated to form an equilibrium. All have equal status. If one pattern within the whole is harmed, everything else within the whole is harmed. If the balance of the planet is disturbed, illness and disaster can result.

NURSING ENVIRONMENTAL ACTION

If we accept this holistic view of a unitary, alive, and interacting environment, what effect might it have on us individually and on our profession? First, we will have a new consciousness and understanding of our planet and our place within it. We will understand our world to be an enormous living, undivided, and interacting organism. We are a part of it, equal to all other parts. Perhaps then we can live in harmony with our world rather than attempting to dominate it. Second, we will understand that any actions that we take individually are globally related and interconnected. Our actions, in turn, affect the universe and the cosmos.

Perceiving the environment holistically in terms of being alive, whole, and interacting can affect the way that we practice nursing. The participants in my focus study understood this concept clearly. They recommended: (a) making the community and broader environment our nursing client, (b) redirecting our nursing activities to the macro-level environment, and (c) moving the profession from oppression to empowerment in order to make the necessary transformations.

When we make the community our nursing client and direct our nursing actions to the community, we will directly address the issue of a toxic dump or a similar threat to health and well-being. Our efforts might prevent many people from getting leukemia. This use of nursing resources is much more effective than taking care of an individual child who has already contracted the disease. Taking action at the community level will be a recognized nursing action.

When we make the planet itself our nursing client, we will take global nursing action. Understanding the interactions between our use of resources and the degradation of the environment will enable us to acquire a global mentality. What we do in our country can gravely affect people in other parts of the world. Their actions, in turn, directly affect us. For instance, the uses of wood products in Western countries have resulted in cutting down the rain forests in developing countries. Disruption and disease in these indigenous cultures and desertification of the rain forests have followed. Desertification, in turn, results in global warming and depletion of the world's oxygen, which directly affects our health. An understanding of these links makes it legitimate to take nursing action in the global arena.

To empower the profession, our actions will need to be informed by our own holistic paradigms of healing and caring. To make the transformations that we need to make, we must incorporate the environmental perspectives discussed in this chapter. As nurses, we will individually, through our nursing organizations, and in partnership with other concerned organizations, enter into the larger global, social, economic, and political arenas of the environment in order to address these and other urgent health-related concerns.

PERSONAL STATEMENT

My interests relating to the environment began as a child, when I went camping and hiking with my family. I discovered a new and marvelous world of plants and animals in their own natural environments, which did not exist in the city of Los Angeles where I grew up. These early interests were rekindled in adulthood, when I again took backpacking and hiking trips. I began to realize that there soon would be no natural areas left in this country. I joined with other members of the Sierra Club, a conservation organization, to work on saving the remaining wilderness areas.

I began to think about the environment in relation to nursing when I entered the nursing doctoral program at the University of San Diego. I found that the idea of environment in the nursing literature was different and more circumscribed than my ideas about environment. I continued to pursue this study and wrote several class papers focused on the environment. My studies culminated with my dissertation research on the topic. During the doctoral program, my environmental perspectives changed from "saving the wilderness" to "saving the planet."

Today, I consider environmental degradation to be the major threat to all living things on our planet. I believed that the nursing profession, with its interest in the health and well-being of humans, is raising its consciousness and going through an exciting environmental paradigm shift, as evidenced by this book. The profession has the potential of being a dynamic and vital force in worldwide environmental efforts. I want to be involved with these endeavors.

REFERENCES

Ames, R. T. (1986). Taoism and the nature of nature. *Environmental Ethics, 8*(4), 317–350.

Anderson, J. M. (1991). Reflexivity in fieldwork: Toward a feminist epistemology. *Image: The Journal of Nursing Scholarship, 23*(2), 115–118.

Bohm, D. (1980). *Wholeness and the implicate order.* London: Routledge & Kegan Paul.

Booth, A. L., & Jacobs, H. M. (1990). Ties that bind: Native American beliefs as a foundation for environmental consciousness. *Environmental Ethics, 12*(1), 27–43.

Callicott, J. B. (1982). Traditional American Indian and Western European attitudes toward nature: An overview. *Environmental Ethics, 4*(4), 293–318.

Chopoorian, T. J. (1986). Reconceptualizing the environment. In P. Moccia (Ed.), *New approaches to theory development* (pp. 39-54). New York: National League for Nursing.

Devall, B., & Sessions, G. (1985). *Deep ecology.* Salt Lake City, UT: Peregrine Smith.

Eisler, R. (1990). The Gaia tradition and the partnership future: An ecofeminist manifesto. In I. Diamond & G. F. Orenstein (Eds.), *Reweaving the world: The emergence of ecofeminism* (pp. 23-34). San Francisco: Sierra Club.

Hughes, J. D. (1982). Gaia: Environmental problems in Chthonic perspective. *Environmental Review, 6*(2), 92-104.

Ip, P. (1983). Taoism and the foundations of environmental ethics. *Environmental Ethics, 3*(3), 335-343.

Kingry, M. J., Tiedje, L. B., & Friedman, L. L. (1990). Focus groups: A research technique for nursing. *Nursing Research, 39*(2), 124-125.

Kleffel, D. (1991). Rethinking the environment as a domain of nursing knowledge. *Advances in Nursing Science, 14*(1), 40-51.

Kleffel, D. (1994). *The environment: Alive, whole, and interacting.* Unpublished doctoral dissertation, University of San Diego, San Diego, CA.

Lovelock, J. E. (1979). *Gaia: A new look at life on earth.* New York: Oxford University Press.

Lovelock, J. E. (1988). *The ages of Gaia: A biography of our living earth.* New York: Norton.

Meleis, A. I. (1991). *Theoretical nursing: Development and progress* (2nd ed.). Philadelphia: Lippincott.

Morgan, D. L. (1988). *Focus groups as qualitative research* (Sage University Paper Series on Qualitative Research Methods, Vol. 16). Newbury Park, CA: Sage.

Naess, A. (1973). The shallow and the deep, long-range ecology movement: A summary. *Inquiry, 16,* 95-100.

Neihardt, J. G. (1931). *Black Elk speaks.* Lincoln NE: University of Nebraska Press.

Nightingale, F. (1969). *Notes on nursing: What it is and what it is not.* New York: Dover. (Original work published in 1860.)

Peerenboom, R. P. (1992). Beyond naturalism: A reconstruction of Taoist environmental ethics. *Environmental Ethics, 13*(1), 3-22.

Strauss, A., & Corbin, J. (1991). *Basics of qualitative research.* Newbury Park, CA: Sage.

Talbot, M. (1991). *The holographic universe.* New York: HarperPerennial.

Warren, K. J. (1987). Feminism and ecology: Making connections. *Environmental Ethics, 9*(1), 3-20.

Wei-Ming, T. (1989). The continuity of being: Chinese visions of nature. In J. B. Callicott & R. T. Ames (Eds.), *Nature in Asian traditions of thought: Essays in environmental philosophy* (pp. 67-78). New York: SUNY Press.

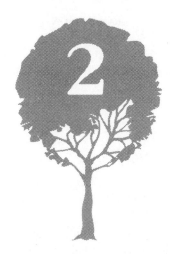

A Frog, a Rock, a Ritual: Myth, Mystery, and Metaphors for an Ecocaring Cosmology in a Universe That Is Turning Over

Jean Watson

LOST MOTHER

This topic begins with a passage written centuries ago by Hildegard of Bingen:

> *The Earth is at the same time Mother. She is the mother of all that is natural, mother of all that is human. She is the Mother of all, for contained in her are the seeds of all. (Hildegard of Bingen, 12th century, quoted in Fox, 1985)*

Did you know that during this century we lost our Mother?
Lost our Mother, you say? How can that be? How do we know this?
(Pearson, 1992).

A Frog

We know because of the frogs!
The frogs, you say?
Yes, the frogs! (Yoffe, 1992)

It started in the vast, pristine wilderness of Colorado, where Dr.
Cynthia Carey, a biologist on the University of Colorado—Boulder
campus discovered that all the frogs for her research were disappearing; they were dying! Their immune systems were collapsing!

The loss of our Mother became more evident when the loss of
the frogs was realized as a phenomenon that was not local to Colorado. It soon became known that even Mark Twain's red-legged
frog, hero of "The Celebrated Jumping Frog of Calaveras County,"
was missing (Yoffe, 1992).

Yes, it's true, and there's more. Even the ". . . Yosemite Toad,
and the Mountain Yellowlegged frog are found in short supply.
And another thing, did you know that Southern California is virtually barren of most of its native frogs? That Canada has lost its

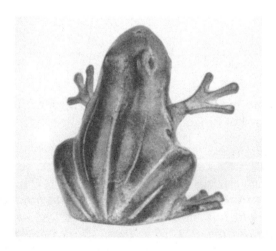

Northern Leopard frog?" Costa Ricans are missing some of their commonly known amphibians, and the same is true in other parts of Central America, South America, Australia, Italy, and England. This has occurred in spite of the fact that, as late as 1977, six new species of frogs were found in Western Australia (Olson, 1984, p. 296).

Actually, it is now documented that the golden toad frog is missing around the globe. Herpetologists, naturalists, and biologists worldwide are pondering the "mysterious silence of the frogs"!

Did you ever consider, however, that frogs are the ideal creature to reflect the health of the environment and our caring/noncaring consciousness? They are a bridge between the aquatic and the terrestrial, the link between fish and reptile. The mediators of the mythic and mystical, they symbolize verdant greenness, power, water, fertility, sustainability; they link water and life with the earth. They have survived 200 million years, existed from the Himalayas to the Sonoran Desert, and outlasted the dinosaurs.

On other levels—environmentally, mythically, and metaphysically—we now can begin to understand: the lowly frog is the medium and the messenger, the Cassandra for our time, signaling the mysterious loss of our Mother. The frogs are telling us about the environment's overall health and our caring/noncaring relationship to Mother Earth.

The silence of the frogs represents the destruction of biological diversity, life's evolution, less flexibility for new food sources, less ability for all to survive, the collapse of the ecosystem. Loss of frogs means loss of what Hildegard of Bingen called *Veriditas*— greening power, lush greening, wetness. Its loss is resulting in shriveled and wilted people and institutions, and the wilting of our Mother. The poignant prophecy from a frog census is that frogs aren't the only creature disappearing; they are only one messenger representing migratory songbirds, rhinoceroses, and other diminishing species. Researchers estimate that one quarter to one half of the earth's species could become extinct in the next 30 years (Yoffe, 1992).

The connection between our Mother and the frog story is that this extinction, unlike the dinosaurs, is the first to be caused by humans (Yoffe, 1992).

Thus, we *have* lost our Mother and our link among humans, nature, and all living things. We now know it because of the frog story. But the frogs are only one story.

A Rock

The Aborigines of Australia tell another story about the loss of our Mother. They say it occurred when the Anglo-Europeans drove a stake into the heart of *Uluru,* Ayer's rock, to accommodate the tourists. The stake was driven into the most sacred site on their earth: the sacred center of their land and their continent. They say that's when the spirits left their Sacred Rock Home and their Mother was lost.

There's another story from the Wongi Tribe of the Aboriginal Dreamtime world, from the outback of Australia. Remember, according to their mythology, the "Aboriginal Dreaming is 'Eternal'— Dreaming is still happening. Their ancestors are still alive today as guardian spirits which are a living part of the rocks, trees, animals, and people. To know their Dreaming, they have only to look, listen and live" (Aboriginal Culture Abroad, 1988, p. 6).

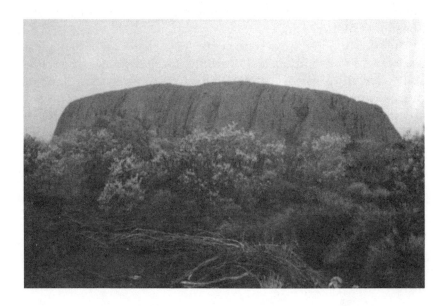

One of their Dreaming stories was told to me by an Elder Aboriginal, and it came out this way:

Dreamtime and Sharing the Tears with the Wongi Tribe of Cundeelee

He said it like this.

It's world behind in Dreamtime.
It's finished, we're free.
The Wongi for Caring
means "sharing the tears."
We want help to get to our nearest place
to find all our relations
to carry on the debate.
How to release the Community
from the State.
The State that denies them the
"time out" they need
to fill up their sorrow
pour out the grief.
The greed of the Country,
the business, the mines
that won't let the people
wail as they need.
When all they ask for is time out
to grieve.
It's so deep, so painful.

They say it all hurts.
They must be alone to properly mourn
Cause our fields are from Dreamtime
that penetrates years
and guides all our people
to bury their fears
to trust one another
and learn to obey
to believe in our sisters and brothers

in spite of their ways.
To wish for them goodness
even when they pray
regardless of memories
and haunting decay.

They sit and they hope
they sleep in the night
beyond all comprehension of
white man's likes.
They watch in the heavens
for the Milky Way paths,
Emu noises and black holes
that quake.
The earth, the water, the birds
and the fowl.
The animals and trees and
certainly the tail of the
lowliest Kangaroo
that shivers and quails.
When all men are gone
according to scale.

We knew it all through hundreds of stories.
Dreamtime continues to wail.
The grief you say is only one tale.

The forebears' Dreamtimes
are mighty and powerful
and all we entail.
The earth is our partner
one whole of this life.
It's sacred to feel
and sinful to fail.

The Dreamtime shows us now never to err
When it comes to uncovering
the Rocks and the soil,

Because of the death and
destruction that's left
in the trail.

Instead of objects and gemstones
and people with dreams
Only death and destruction
Youla—*I mean*
Even the name change
to Yolaria—
Can't change the tune
That's played for Mankind
once the notes are produced.

So leave it alone, don't tamper with fate
The Uranium's a hate of the whole human race,
Except for the miners and sharers of great
The Dreamers of Visions
for money and fame;
For you see,
rights and fights
and claims are at stake.

But listen to wisdom, to time,
and my stories of late
That have been told by the
Dreamtime and hold us
awake.

If only we hear the children
and the chants in the night,
The stars in the heavens
That show us what's right
The soul's reawakening will
come in the night
If you listen to Dreamtime
before all goes quiet.
(Watson, 1988, pp. 97-99; reprinted with permission of the
author)

From 12th-century scientist, mystic, and saint Hildegard of Bingen to indigenous peoples through thousands of years, we hear the same story.

Contemporary writers, scientists, philosophers, and historians alike tell us still one more story about losing our Mother. During this so-called modern era of humankind, there is knowledge that has been systematically excluded from the human consciousness. In this postmodern time, the modern era has left us with a crisis in the rituals and myths that connect us with our Mother and our earthly ties (Smith, 1982).

They say *that* is how we lost our Mother, by excluding her from our consciousness, our knowledge, our worship, our myths, our rituals—indeed, our living—and now our very existence is at stake. All because of a frog and a rock and a few lost rituals.

But frogs are ugly and rocks are worthless; why do we need them to have our Mother Earth? And rituals are for pagans and witches, and are meaningless acts. And for that matter, why do we even need our Mother? We, who are adults in a world and universe of our own, don't need anything. We have dominion over all the lowly rocks and stones and frogs as well as the sun, the moon, and the stars.

But Annie Dillard's (1977, 1982) refrain remains, reminding us: "It is all, God help us, a matter of Rocks. The Rocks shape life like hands around swelling dough" (p. 127).

And T. S. Eliot's *The Waste Land* (1988/1919) sings out to us:

. . . If there were water
And no rock
If there were rock
And also water
And water . . . .

The rock and water merged for Maclean (1976) as he lamented: "Eventually, all things merge into one and A River Runs Through It . . . and runs over rocks from the basement of time. . . . Under the Rocks are the words, and some of the words are theirs" [the Rocks']. And through it all, "I am haunted by water . . ." (p. 76).

So, now—somewhere deep inside, we know there is a new moon rising; we are leaving the ancient Mayan calendar of pisces after 2,000 years—a time of advances, industrialization, science, and technology, but also a time of wars, violence, power over others and over our Mother (Arguelles, 1984).

We know it is time

We can wait no longer.

We now must move to embrace the mystery—the eternal source of wisdom full of truths and myths to live by in harmony with self, all our relations, the planet to consider the dark mystery of silence where the frogs live and seek light and energy from the rocks and water and other living things.

And besides: have you not heard?

The universe is turning over! . . . This very moment!?

Can you *feel it? Hear it?* The frogs are still croaking, even while becoming extinct.

And, do you know, the wind is blowing from the four sacred corners of the earth, North-South-East-West, and the Goddess is emerging from the dark side of the moon? Annie Dillard (1982) knows someone who is teaching a stone to *talk,* this moment; an Aboriginal woman or Maori or American Indian is remembering the teaching stones of ancestors to keep them connected with our Mother. Somewhere out there right now, someone of Celtic lore is listening to talking trees. Furthermore, Hopi Indian Earth Corn Spirits—*Corn Mother herself*—is feeding the body and spirit of "all my relations." Being harvested as a sacred gift from our Mother—symbol of new life, of resurrection, awakening, fertility, and germination.

A Ritual

So now do you know? About the universe turning? If so, we can recreate meaningful rituals to bring light to the dark side—the mystery side—of the universe, and coparticipate in this cosmic turn of the universe. If so, then we can now retell the ritual story.

The ritual story began in Sweden, the land of the dark, the land of the north—the direction of the mystery—where the North Star

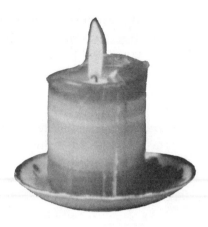

is the center around which skies revolve. It is the site of the Arctic Circle—the home of ancients. This is the land where people hold wisdom in their heart and offer a great deal of reverence to the light; they pay attention to the light–dark cycle. This is especially true in the brief hours of sunlight they have during the winter months. They make great use of candles, of light, and of life's living in general. During my time there and in other Scandinavian countries, they almost always had candlelight during my talks and seminars. Upon my return to Colorado, in 1992, I recreated the candle experience with a group of doctoral students from throughout North America. At the end of the five-day seminar, every student had independently bought a candle and lit it from the original candle, now in the Center for Human Caring. The students then took their own candles and their symbolic light back to their homes and places of study and practice, to pass on the light of nursing' reawakening. One of the students called it, metaphorically and symbolically, the Goddess candle, the feminine spirit energy of nursing being rekindled. Nurses from around the world have told me they see the Center as a place that holds the light for nursing's crossing into the next century and relighting the lamp. I have repeated this candle ritual of passing on the light of caring with nurses in every place I have been since—New Zealand, Australia, the United Kingdom, Canada, and throughout the United States.

Recreating meaningful rituals helps us to reconnect, allowing for new beginnings and celebrations of continuity, as well as endings, mergings, cycles, and healings. A ritual of light helps us to touch our heritage; it symbolizes the birth of a new wholeness emerging. As Joseph Campbell and others say, rituals allow us to enter a timeless world; to give new form to our existence; to enter a place, often unremembered, that still surrounds us, just beyond our ordinary reach (Beck & Metrick, 1990, p. iii).

Fox (1985) says we need a revolution in rituals to help us pass on our values and meanings to the next generation. The modern world has a poverty and crisis of rituals, so I now pass on the ritual of light. Let us relight the symbolic lamp of nursing and keep its energy moving and uninterrupted as it extends to nurses and nursing around the world, awakening to and honoring their heritage light, the symbolic Nightingale lamp, and passing it on.

I am recalling the teachings of Brooke Medicine Eagle (1993), who said: "If we stand in the light, the light is shed on 10,000" (p. 8). American Indians advise us to make an act of power with our ritual, with our personal work as well as our professional work; to make an act of beauty wherever we are. Nightingale reminded us that, every day, a patient should have something beautiful to look at. This passing of the light of nursing's caring consciousness is my act of power and beauty for myself, for us, for nursing, and for our Mother.

Now that *you* are part of the frog, the rock, and the ritual story, you are part of the universe that is turning over—a contributor to the turning of the universe.

There is a new morning, an entering into the mystery, myth, and metaphors of the light, away from the shadow sleep. The mist of Avalon is lifting; the rock-dead universe is being replaced with a Planet Earth ascending, this moment—full of light, of living rocks and frogs, corn, trees, and rivers. Perhaps as we approach this other side of the universe, we can begin to understand Maya Angelou's (1993) chant of morning, which captures the essence of the cosmic tree of life.

A CHANT OF MORNING

Maya Angelou's (1993) chant: "On the Pulse of Morning" reconnects us with our light, our ancient heritage, and our archetypal ties with this "green ball which floats us" as she helps us remember—a rock, a river, a tree:

> *As we hear the Rock cry out to come and stand on its back*
> *and face our distant destiny; imploring us to not hide our*
> *face, to come to my Riverside, to sing the songs the Creator*
> *gave to me when I and Tree and Rock were one. Reminding*
> *us still that . . . . There is a true yearning to respond to "The*
> *singing River and wise Rock," to have a reunion with all my*
> *relations.*
> *They all hear*
> *The speaking of the Tree . . .*
> *Speaks to humankind today. Come*
> *to me here beside the River . . .*
> *Here root yourselves beside me. I am that*
> *Tree planted by the River, [that Rock] which will not be*
> *moved.*

ANGELS AND ALL LIVING THINGS

Did you not know that in this chant of the morning in a universe that is turning over we can commune with angels? Did you know that all indigenous people, that transcendental poets, philosophers, scientists, theologians, and mystics alike, that Emerson, Thoreau, Whitehead, and Chardin all chanted the same liberating song line as Angelou about "all our relations with all living things" toward our emancipation and evolution with the planet?

Yes, the universe *is* turning over; the living earth is issuing an evocation from the farthest reaches of infinity. Desperate earthlings of the past, those afflicted with the shadow condition of "Maximum Human-centered Commercial and Machine Entropy" (adapted from Arguelles, 1984, p. 147) are being scattered to the universe and being replaced by guardians—angels, in fact, of aesthetic, mythic, and spiritual unification of human and planetary evolution.

Annie Dillard actually sighted these guardian angels—"in those hills!" "[T]housands of spirits, . . . in fact, almost discernable to the eye and whirling . . . ." If pressed, the angel sightings were "three or four feet from the ground . . . their beauty unspeakable." So indeed, she witnessed, "there *are* angels in those fields and I presume in *all* fields, and everywhere else" (Dillard, 1982, pp. 137–138).

I even sighted them myself only recently, Druidlike angels, dancing on the walls of a 14th-century Danish church in Sweden. Imagine, women too; women angels dancing on the ancient church ceilings!

You probably did not know that Emerson's angels preceded Annie's angels in the hills, but came much later than the Danish church angels. His angels were not only guardians, but actually creators of this universe:

> *What angels invented these splendid ornaments, these rich conveniences, this ocean of air above, this ocean of water beneath, this firmament of earth between? This zodiac of lights, this tent of dropping clouds, this striped coat of climates, this fourfold year? Beasts, fire, water, stones, and corn serve us. The field is at once our floor, our work yard, our playground, our garden and our bed. (Emerson, 1982, p. 40)*

Is it possible that there is a Goddess at work in this miraculous universe which is turning over? Are *you* able to locate yourself with the original haunting, elemental, divine, jeweled patterns of life itself? Can you fathom the human consciousness of a universal reflective soul within or behind your individual life, wherein, as in a firmament, the natures of caring and love arise and shine as the jewel that holds the infinite facets and reflects all of the other jewels and their relations. All of this reminds us: "[T]hat which intellectually considered we call Reason, considered in relation to nature, we call Spirit. Spirit is the Creator. Spirit hath life in itself" (Emerson, 1982, p. 49).

Do you agree with Emerson (1982/1936) that ". . . the universe is composed of Nature and the Soul" (p. 36)? "That nature is the symbol of spirit" (p. 48) and that spirit—breath, life, energy; fire, air, water, rock, sky, and earth itself—are part of one Great Spirit? Do you believe that the Goddess creator, like creation, is at the core of life, and is about relation, and:

> *All our relations . . . implying all beings, all things, the ones we see and the ones we do not; the whirling galaxies and the*

*wild suns, the black holes and the microorganisms, the trees
and the stars, the fish and the flowers and the rocks, the
birthing of children. Creation is all space, all time—all
things past, present, and future. (Fox, 1991, pp. 8-9)*

Can you consider a place that is not human-centered; where, instead, the human is decentered and takes its place in the context of a living cosmology, perhaps what I would call a living-caring cosmology that makes room for our Great Mother, the giver of life and creator of all? There would be a hint of worship of the Goddess of nature and spirituality I saw uncovered on the ancient Celtic ceilings.

Can we acknowledge the ancient traditions of the Earth—vegetation, fire, birds, and water—equated with the female? Indeed, most tribes and cultures throughout time have carried a female persona and believe the cosmos is held together in a womblike structure, à la Hildegard of Bingen.

To consider a living-caring cosmology in this turning universe, one may wish to concur with Emerson (1982/1936): "Nature refers to essences unchanged by human: space, the air, the river, [the rock, the frog], the leaf, the corn, the stars" (p. 36).

One would need to ask, as does Emerson (1982/1936): "Do you delight with the fields and woods"? Do you believe Emerson's notion that there is "an occult relation between human and the vegetable"? That, in their midst, he discovered, "I am not alone and unacknowledged. They nod to me, and I to them" (p. 39)?

Could you then believe in Living Earth stories and myths such as I have heard and read and seen at the Findhorn Community, located at a prehistoric site of northernmost Scotland? This oldest (30 years old) successful commune in the world has a vision for an emerging planetary family (Findhorn Community Foundation, 1980). The vision was created through communicating in the manner of Emerson's occult human-vegetable relations—those elemental forces and divine patterns that acknowledged to the founders that they were not alone and unacknowledged. They and the flowers and vegetables mutually nodded to each other and they both prospered.

From this other side of the turning universe, can you begin to understand why over 60 percent of Norwegians and other

Scandinavians living in deeply natural surroundings reportedly believe in trolls, fairies, and elemental forces? Or why a colleague-friend in Sweden wrote me that she prefers to call Christmas by its ancient pre-Christian name, *Jul,* meaning the light in the dark, the Gaia creation?

I suspect that, by now, you begin to see:

- Why deeply ethical environmental lawyers say that trees and streams have rights of their own and that to alter the natural flow of the river would cut our Mother Earth off from the very source of life itself. We, like Maclean, are and need to be "haunted by water."

- Why Naturalists report that "when we explore the . . . provision that has been made for our support and delight on this green ball which floats us through the heaven, . . . the misery of the human appears like childish petulance" (Emerson, 1982, p. 40).

- Why environmentalists and naturalists are pointing out that, because economists have not even put our Mother Earth into the calculation of cost, our Mother gets lost and is not considered; the economists have seen nothing wrong in destruction and uncontrolled growth, in silencing the frogs and losing our Mother. They also see nothing amiss in leaving caring for self and Mother out of the health/societal equation.

But that is the other side of the universe—the side that we are leaving behind.

From this side of the universe, you can perhaps better grasp why Pele, the Volcano goddess—myth of Hawaii, has to erupt, allowing her lava to flow and spread, uninterrupted, to the sea—in search of all her children, to heal the pain they have caused.

As this universe turns, and as we see it from this side, perhaps we can glimpse the approaching global revolution necessary to place us on a firm footing with the evolutionary process.

Did you know that this universe turning is removing us from the shadow, which is antiquated, toward a new light, helping us to discard a consciousness no longer attuned to the times? As José Arguelles put it (1984), we now have an incentive to "cross the great water," to approach the metaphoric bridge that spans troubled and turbulent waters and leads to either human and planetary demise or human transformation.

The Mayan and Aztec calendars saw this turning as a fire in the lake which is setting the calendar of humankind in order; a turn allowing the four seasons and sacred scattered energies of the universe to come back together to complete themselves, to make us whole again. We now see more clearly—the leave-taking of the age of pisces of this Mayan calendar—into an earth ascending spirit filled with life, creativity, nurturing—a caring cosmology (Arguelles, 1984).

As Elise Boulding (1989), sociologist, Quaker, and peace studies scholar, calls out to us with her chant:

We are standing on the threshold of the cosmos, and we do not know who we are. Either we discover our identity and move into a new dimension [the turning of the universe] of spiritual existence, along with our technical conquests of time and space, or we shrink back into substance [Hildegard's wilting and shriveling of people and institutions] as a race of well-trained clerical assistants, timidly feeding data into gigantic computers to find out what to do next. Who is taking "Time Out" to probe for new dimensions that will open up a way of life not now imagined? Who is dreaming dreams? Who is seeing visions? [and angels?] Where are they? (p. 26)

Can *we* pause to comprehend that we are part of the universe turning, ushering in one of these seasonal ancient calendar revolutions? Do we know that this is a turning by attunement, a harmonizing of the heavens and earth, an appeasement of the gods and goddesses of the universe?

SOPHIA, GAIA, THE MOTHER GODDESS

From this threshold of the cosmos we hear in the distance Sophia, Mother Earth Goddess, the emergent Gaia, singing to us, both scientifically and poetically, that the Living Earth has a soul. We *are* a self-organizing universe. There *is* an inner radiance and life spirit–energy that is protected and blessed by all the indigenous peoples of the world and *all* our relations. The tradition of Sophia is both mystical and cosmological: "Even in the biblical literature, the mind is personified as a woman who undergirds and permeates all things. She brings order from chaos. She carries the fruit of awe and wonder" (Fox, 1991, p. 64). We understand that the material world and the spiritual world are only a sacred reflection of the universe, within and without, that must be experienced.

Are you aware that we can make and we are making new environmental caring connections, even in this brief moment of coming together? Can you consider that we are helping to heal the severance between mind and matter, between nature and life, between earth and the celestial, between biota and soul?

THE SACRED DIRECTIONS OF THE
TURNING OF THE WHEEL

Come along with me to create spaces for the soul of humankind and Mother Earth by remembering the elemental and divine patterns of this life and our original relationship with the earth forces. Take four last turns with me on the indigenous wheel of life. Come with me into the four sacred directions of the universe as we reclaim our relations with all the elemental forces, with all our relations, at all points in the universe.

- North reconnects us to the *rock,* the home of the ancients. This is the most powerful direction, the direction of the mystery, the dark, the northern regions where the sun never reaches; the land of the midnight sun and of winter; the place of silence and power, a place to be still and listen. Listen to the turning of the wheel as the skies revolve around the North Star, which is the center of the wheel and the center of the cycle that represents Earth and wisdom.

  Corn stands for Earth itself; it stands for the body, which brings forth seed; for germination, the vegetables, and holy sustenance of all living things. Corn Earth Mother represents spirit, or maize—the sacred food, the gift of life. North is the physical body and our embodied Mother, now requiring a sacred covenant to cherish her.

- South reconnects us with the *ritual* of life; it corresponds to the element *fire,* to energy, spirit, the noontime, summertime. South is related to wonder, to innocence; it brings forth the quality of our will; it is a teacher of trust. It also stands for the light and for passing on the light of our caring energy, our passion—experienced through a reenactment of ritual.

- East reconnects us with the metaphorical *angels;* it too brings illumination; a quest for visionary truth. East corresponds with the elemental force of *air;* it is associated with the lightness of Being—the power to know; the dawn of morning, springtime. East is our breath, our life force, the expansion-contraction, inspiring-expiring, rising-falling cycle of breath of the universe.

- West finally brings us full-circle on the wheel of life and reconnects us with the *frog,* the mythic and mystical creature that has been mysteriously silenced and is disappearing, but now can be rediscovered. West symbolizes our intuition and emotions; it corresponds to *water,* twilight, autumn, the sea, sea serpents, fish, dolphins. It calls forth power to dare, to have courage and face our deepest feelings. Water and the west represent our source, the cleansing of the body and soul. They are the rain that feeds the plant and sustains us.

Who looks upon a river in a meditative hour and is not reminded of the flux of all things? Throw a stone into the stream, and the circles that propagate themselves are the beautiful type of all influence. (Emerson, 1982, p. 49)

West, the sacred direction, captures the concentric circles of caring from self to the universe, like the stone in the water or the Chambered Nautilus, which propagates the circles into infinity.

CONCENTRIC CIRCLES OF COSMIC CARING

This cycle of the four sacred directions, the turning of the cosmic wheel of infinity, is captured by the poets:

The wind sows the seed; the sun evaporates the sea; the wind blows the vapor to the field; the ice, on the other side of the planet, condenses rain on this; the rain feeds the plant; the plant feeds the animal; and thus the endless circulations of the divine charity [of caring cosmology] nourish us. (Emerson, 1982/1936, p. 41)

This caring circle of infinity can be experienced by the "centering silence" of presencing ourselves to this moment in the universe. We must rejoin ourselves, individually and collectively, with a caring consciousness, a living cosmology that unites and attunes scientific forces with the myth, mystery, and metaphor of the mythic and mystical forces that reside on this other side of the universe that is continually turning over.

The last step is crossing the internal bridge of our consciousness and entering into this *living caring cosmology for our Lost Mother.* As Arguelles (1984) reminded us: We are going to make it across the bridge and bridge the mysterious silence between worlds and time—or we are not going to make it. This is a time to put our energy together in the light to make a difference.

THE PERSONAL/COSMIC CARING AND TURNING

Finally, with the crossover, after having metaphorically and symbolically communed with scientists, naturalists, mystics, and angels, we now experience one last turn of the great wheel that has moved through the four sacred directions. This last turn into infinity was anticipated by the cosmic mandela of Hildegard of Bingen in the 12th century. It now offers a promise of a new moon and a new tomorrow:

When we inhale the air and let the wind caress our face and body;
When we drink of water as the holy source, tune our rhythm to its flow—to cleanse, purify, nourish, rejoice;
When we feel the fire of our passion, recreate our rituals, channel its
light and heat to protect our shadow of winter cold;
When we ingest the corn as Mother's sacred gift of sustenance;
Then we will teach a stone to speak and a tree to talk;
And when the day is done, and we stand peacefully with this Living
Earth—this hallowed piece of land on the planet
This "Holy but Firm" *site—*
When we are at one with self and "all our relations"
then we too will know what Emerson, Dillard, mystics, saints, and
scientists already know—
That we are one and the same.

But once again, when we pause—to be still—
To be Holy but Firm, to take it all in,
When we are able to dwell, even briefly, in that space, that space of
pulse, of pause between inspiring-expiring; between contracting-
expanding; rising and falling; between destroying-creating;
When we are able to hold all of the universe in that holy, quiet, still
moment;

Then, in the quiet when we will have entered the sacred space:
We *will hear the frogs; see the angels.*
But then—*just* then, *and only then—in that quiet space when* you *hear*
the frogs, will you *too KNOW?*

PERSONAL STATEMENT

We breathe in our environments and they come into us, just as the air we breathe, thus consideration of the environment is as critical as consideration of breathing and the breath of life. For, you see, environment in its fullest sense is symbolized by nature and nature is the symbol for life's spirit, connecting us and all that we breathe in together. Without attending to the environment, reconnecting with environment and nature, we now see, at this turn of the 20th century, that we cannot survive on planet Earth, without radical attention to our environment.

Environment to me is as necessary for the soul as the body. I need places for my soul and I wither in space that is sterile and institutional. That is why I work very hard to pay attention to environment, even in the midst of harsh spaces where we often find ourselves in the world of nursing and educational and practice settings.

As we see the environment being destroyed, we are all awakening to the reality that we are all keepers of the environment and nature, lest we see the demise of life as we know it.

Personally, nature, the mountains, and the sea are my sacred environmental spaces; they restore and soothe; they provide life energy itself for me personally, as they also connect me with all living things. Nature is my solace—my soul care that I seek and need on a regular basis. If I lose touch with nature, I lose touch with self and my soul and life spirit. In hiking into the mountain park, which is two blocks from my home, whether alone on the Sea of Cortez in Mexico or another part of the world, nature calls me to gain my balance and reconnect with my deepest self.

In my home in Boulder, Colorado, I seek this alone time. I sometimes sit on a special rock that faces the Flatiron Mountain formation and meditate and journal. Other times I sit quietly by the mountain stream which is the site of the snow run-off and quietly watch and listen to the sounds of the birds, the wind, and the running water, all reminding me of the passing of all things, the life energy run-off that keeps all things flowing with the river of time, like life itself.

So, whether on a snowcapped mountain, hiking on Bald mountain, communicating with my gargoyle tree, the one that is old and wise and gnarled, or sitting alone in my yard with its big trees and bird life, I am called to nature, just as surely as are the birds. Nature is my art and my spirit for life's livings and life's beauty.

REFERENCES

Aboriginal Culture Abroad. (1988). *The teaching stones of the outcast tribe.* Western Australia: Aboriginal Culture Abroad Publishing, Ltd.

Angelou, M. (1993, January 20). *On the pulse of morning.* Inaugural Poem. Inauguration of President Bill Clinton, Washington, DC.

Arguelles, J. (1984). *Earth ascending: An illustrated treatise on laws governing whole systems.* Boulder, CO: Shambhala Press.

Beck, R., & Metrick, S. (1990). *The art of ritual.* Berkeley, CA: Celestial Arts.

Boulding, E. (1989). *One small plot of heaven: Reflections on family life by a Quaker sociologist.* Wallingford, PA: Pendel Hill Publishing.

Brooke Medicine Eagle. (1993). The path of sacred ecology. (Interview by Jed Swift.) *The Monthly Newspaper of the Rocky Mountain Spiritual Emergence Network, 5*(2), 1.

Dillard, A. (1977). *Holy the firm.* New York: Harper & Row Publishing.

Dillard, A. (1982). *Teaching a stone to talk.* New York: Perennial Library.

Eliot, T. S. (1983). The waste land. In *The Norton Anthology of Poetry* (3rd ed.), p. 1009. New York: Norton. (Original work published in 1919.)

Emerson, R. W. (1982/1936). *Selected essays.* New York: Penguin Books.

Findhorn Community Foundation. (1980). *Faces of Findhorn.* New York: Harper & Row. (Original work published 1936).

Fox, M. (1985). *Illumination of Hildegard of Bingen.* Santa Fe, NM: Bean & Co.

Fox, M. (1991). *Creation spirituality.* San Francisco, CA: Harper & Row.

Maclean, N. (1976). *A river runs through it.* Chicago: University of Chicago Press.

Pearson, C. L. (1992). *Mother wove the morning.* Walnut Creek, CA: Pearson Publishing.

Smith, H. (1982). *Beyond the post-modern mind.* London: Theosophical Publishing House.

Watson, J. (1988). *Nursing: Human science and human care.* New York: National League for Nursing.

Yoffe, E. (1992, September 13). Silence of the frogs. *The New York Times Magazine,* 36–39, 64–66, 76.

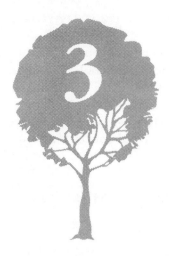

Nightingale, Nursing, and the Ecofeminists

Robert C. Schultz and Phyllis R. Schultz

INTRODUCTION

We began our investigation by exploring the scholarly literature to locate similarities and dissimilarities between Florence Nightingale's thoughts on "nature" and "environment" and those of late 20th-century ecofeminists. We found that many of her ideas on these topics were contained in the long-standing correspondence between Nightingale and Benjamin Jowett, the classicist–philosopher whose translations of Plato were standard texts for many generations of 19th- and 20th-century students of ancient Greek philosophy. Thus, we began by contrasting 19th-century mechanistic notions of nature and environment to contemporary ecofeminist perspectives. Then we located Nightingale's thought within this comparative framework, in an effort to estimate the theoretical distance between her and her professional descendants at the 1993 Boca Raton conference. Our speculations on this question were presented in an "overheard heavenly conversation" between Nightingale and Jowett, which forms the bulk of the chapter that follows. But first we offer a compressed and schematized review of some background concepts and information.

CONCEPTUAL BACKGROUND

Ecofeminism is a complex and dynamic movement of thought. But its rudiments may be identified, drawing on a summary offered by environmental philosopher Max Oelschlaeger (1991):

1. The domination of nature and of women is linked.
2. Earth is our nurturing home and should be revered.
3. Culture–nature, human–nonhuman, and male–female are not superior–inferior pairs.
4. Androcentric concepts, values, and institutions are hurtful to the Earth.
5. Androcentrism must be eradicated if Earth is to be restored. (p. 310)

This ecofeminist understanding of reality stands in sharp contrast to the mechanistic view of nature that emerged in Europe between 1500 and 1700 and has been summarized by Merchant (1989):

1. Our knowledge of nature is certain and consistent.
2. Mathematical laws, not organic processes, govern nature.
3. Force is external to matter; matter is dead stuff.
4. Change is merely rearrangement of particles (images of acorns becoming oaks or babies maturing into adults are misleading).
5. Nature, being dead, may be manipulated and used as resources for human purposes. (pp. 102–103)

Mechanism as a view of nature implies a corresponding methodology for gaining knowledge (Merchant, 1989):

1. Problems are broken into isolated parts and studied/solved apart from each other and the environment.
2. Observations, experiments, and generalizations are hierarchical.
3. Environmental consequences of synthetic products (e.g., pollution) are not important to study.
4. Human consequences of artificial environments (e.g., stress) are not important to study.
5. Following Francis Bacon, we study nature to enlarge human dominance. (pp. 182, 186)

The contrasting methodology for the holistic, or organic, understanding of the ecofeminists may be roughly summarized as follows (Merchant, 1989):

1. Processes are cyclical; to study nature is to study what is active and alive.
2. Wholes collapse if any element is removed for study or some other purpose; elements are defined by their wholes.
3. Parts and wholes are in dialectical, or interactive, relationships.
4. The challenge of ecology is to study nature holistically. (p. 293)

For the present inquiry, where do we locate Florence Nightingale in relation to these contrasting worldviews and methodologies? A review of her own writings and of the secondary literature offers a mixed picture. On the one hand, there is clear evidence of her commitment to the mechanistic, positivist perspectives of her day:

1. Nightingale thought of nature as (God's) laws. (Boyd, 1982, p. 206)

2. Statistical formulation of these laws was her passion; statistics revealed "the character of God." (Cook, 1913, vol. I, p. 480; vol. II, pp. 395–396)

3. Nightingale greatly admired John Stuart Mill's "methods," that is, his rules for the scientific investigation of causal relationships. (Cook, 1913, vol. II, p. 221)

4. "Her empiricism, her love of science, her faith in logic, and her rejection of a supernatural basis for religion all put her in the positivist tradition." (Boyd, 1982, p. 203)

On the other hand, Nightingale's disposition had what might with good reason be thought of as a "postmechanistic" side:

1. Nightingale was against materialism. (see, for example, her letter to Jowett, October 3, 1871, in Quinn & Prest, 1987, p. 220)

2. Nightingale's God-as-Law was also a Lawgiver, a "person." (Cook, 1913, vol. II, pp. 218–219)

3. Nightingale's God was a spirit, "a living thought, feeling, purpose, residing in a conscious being." (Boyd, 1982, p. 206)

4. Nightingale understood herself to be a mystical experiencer of God (Cook, 1913, vol. II, pp. 231–235, 366), in addition to being a statistical recorder of the results of God's laws.

How can this "mixed picture" of Florence Nightingale's intellectual and spiritual being be given some coherence, without overriding the historical evidence? To answer this question, as well as to give a livelier and more personable representation of the founder of modern nursing science and practice, we have chosen to adopt the ancient gambit of a dramatization. We hope that readers will find in the dialogue that follows an account sufficiently anchored in the historical record to be a reliable guide to Nightingale's thought. (We have included some source citations to that end.) At the same time, we have risked a speculative synthesis that we hope will have at least heuristic value for connecting the concerns of their "founding mother" to those of contemporary nursing professionals interested in such basic notions as nature and environment.

A HEAVENLY CONVERSATION

PLACE: Heaven

TIME: March 1993, during the Boca Raton conference on nursing and the environment

CHARACTERS: Benjamin Jowett ("Mr. J"). Florence Nightingale's longtime friend and confidant; a celebrated Plato scholar and sometime Master of Balliol College, Oxford. Jowett had been a regular correspondent of Nightingale for 32 years, beginning in 1860.

              Florence Nightingale ("Miss N"). The "lady of the lamp" was a highly educated woman and the author of some 200 publications and 12,000 letters. She was in active contact with many of the prominent intellectual and political figures in Victorian England, in spite of her reclusive life-style.

MR. J: *(looking up from his writing table)* Well, Miss Nightingale, you've caught me working at my infernal—I mean, eternal—revisions of one of my Plato translations. Remember this passage in the Theatetus where Socrates compares his drawing out of conceptual truths to his mother's midwifery?

MISS N: *(an amused smile crosses her face as she reminisces)* Mr. Jowett, can you have forgotten that I once corrected your Greek in that translation? It was not long after that, I think, that you called me the best critic you'd ever had. And later, I dedicated my *Notes on Lying-In Institutions* [Nightingale, 1871] "to the shade of Socrates' mother."

MR. J: Indeed—I do remember now. And I recall, too, the letter in which you said you were "scandalized" at my "materialistic" reading of Plato, and at Plato's and my neglect of the mental and spiritual aspects of social reality. "I shall shut up you *and* Plato," you wrote, "for a hundred years' punishment in another world till you have both obtained clearer views" [Quinn & Prest, 1987, p. 220]. Think of it: a clean-out-the-gutters realist like you calling the ancient Father of the Forms *and* an Oxford don materialists—both of us in the same breath!!

MISS N: I did like to speak my mind, didn't I—once I'd got it made up, at any rate. I remember saying once that the words "I don't know" were the most insipid and detestable three words in the Queen's English.

MR. J: Do you still think that, Miss Nightingale?

MISS N: Funny you should ask that, Mr. Jowett, because I caught myself using those very words just the other day. There was a nursing conference in Boca Raton— a resort place by the sea in the United States. The nurses were busily talking to one another about the meaning of environment as a nursing concept. And some of them said they were in danger of being defined by their past as members of the nursing profession I founded.

MR. J: Did you disagree with their statistical findings?

MISS N: *(mildly excited and perhaps a little annoyed)* Well, it wasn't very statistical at all, Mr. Jowett! That's part of my puzzlement. They were talking about the agony of the planet, and about kissing the Earth, about healing the planet and ecocaring, and the Earth's four directions, and shamanism, and the med'cine wheel, and holism, and the Gaia hypothesis. They spoke of qualitative research, and feminist methodologies. And then they talked not just of feminism, but of *eco*feminism. The feminism I understand, of course—tho' I sometimes wish they'd stop blathering on about their rights and just get to doing what they can perfectly well do as women [Nightingale, 1859, p. 76]. But the *eco*feminism is something about the earth being exploited and degraded just as women have been. And I just don't know what to make of it all, Mr. Jowett . . . .

MR. J: *(turning reflective)* My dear Miss Nightingale, it's 100 years since you and I both were alive on the earth. The strangeness of some of those ideas probably reflects changes to the earth's environment since I died in 1893, and you in 1910. Pollution, consumption of non-renewable resources, population doubling-times down to 30 or 25 years in places, the spoiling of land and water, mountains of lethal hazardous wastes, ozone depletion, greenhouse warming—and the list goes on: they've got a crisis on their hands that far eclipses our Victorian environmental carelessness—Charles Dickens' Satanic Mills, and all that. But it sounds like the nurses are beginning to look at these large-scale health threats the way you looked years ago at dangers posed by stale air and filthy hospital environments that killed your patients.

Miss N: It's "clients" now, Mr. Jowett. Their way of not letting the sick get too passive. *That* idea's not so strange to me. . . . Perhaps they *are* applying my old concerns about environments on a larger scale. And I see some other connections to my way of thinking, too. Some nurse-scholars still think of nature as a mechanism and study it statistically. And those who don't, at least value careful observations and rigorous thinking as critical to good nursing research and practice.

Mr. J: But can you connect their talk of holism and Gaia with the religious discussions you and I used to have back in the '60s and '70s?

Miss N: Now you're getting to the part I *really* don't know about. I sometimes think I *do* see connections. But then some of the terminology they use leaves me completely cold. *We* talked of God as a stern but loving Father who *created the organisms of the natural order,* but *they* seem to think of all of nature as *itself* a living organism. And for some of them, it's a feminine organism—there's a lot of talk about "Mother" Nature.

Mr. J: Hm . . . I see why it's confusing. Because one could emphasize the commonalities, and note that they, like we, call for reverence toward a deserving and immensely powerful parent. Or one could emphasize the differences—like between masculine governance by a transcendent God who has instituted fixed laws on the one side; and, on the other side, feminine caring, and reverence for nature itself—excuse me, *her*self— as a changing, organic whole.

MISS N: That's it, Mr. Jowett. The differences between their thinking and ours make me wonder how long they'll be able to think of me as their "founding mother." And I worry, too, about how I could function with these new-style nurses in a practical setting. They'd proba- bly call my management style "masculine gover- nance," and invite me to sit down in a circle with them and all share our personal *feelings* about how to run the wards. *(she rolls her eyes upward)* That gives me the shivers! . . . On the other hand, I'm not altogether put off by their talk of spirit and spirituality. I wonder if they remember how I said "The primary fact in reli- gion seems to be the existence of an omnipotent spirit of love and wisdom" [quoted in Boyd, 1982, p. 206], and how I defined "spirit" as "a living thought, feel- ing, purpose, residing in a conscious being" [Boyd, 1982, p. 206]. *(she looks at Mr. J. earnestly)* Do you think, Mr. Jowett, that it comes down to me or them, or could some synthesis be articulated to include both my thought and theirs?

MR. J: Now *there's* an interesting question, Miss Nightingale. As you know, my Greek friends, especially Aristotle, were pretty firm about their dualism. Nowadays, I sup- pose it would be called binary rationality—either God is *Creator* or God is *Nature,* one or the other; either masculine or feminine—you know. But then Hegel, our German contemporary, attracted a lot of attention, with his dialectical scheme for overcoming contra- dictory ideas to save the best of both sides. So maybe there's some way to bridge the contradictions . . . to save the best of your insights about the environments of patients—sorry, clients—and about scientific method, nature, and spirit, and then to connect them to these ecofeminist interpretations.

Miss N: Thank you for reminding me of dialectic. Because that reminds me of a more recent scheme that might help. This one is called "process science," and comes from a writer named David Bohm. He holds that:

> . . . *instead of starting with parts as primary and building up wholes as secondary phenomena, a physics is needed that starts with undivided, multidimensional wholeness (a flow of energy called the holomovement) and derives the three-dimensional world of classical mechanics as a secondary phenomenon. The* explicate *order of the classical world* in which we live *unfolds from the* implicate *order contained in the* underlying flow of energy. *(quoted in Merchant, 1989, p. xvii)*

Mr. J: *(his intellect fully engaged now)* That's pretty heady stuff, Miss Nightingale, for a couple of Victorians like us. An explicate order and an implicate order . . . . But I think I see the key idea—it's like an island in a larger sea. Like that "tight little island" we lived our earthly lives on, set in a surrounding sea that represents a larger but less well understood order: an explicate order within the larger implicate order.

Miss N: Yes. And the point of the image is to allow that *both* the island *and* the sea are real. The goal is to avoid getting trapped in either–or choices, like "either England is real or the sea is real," or "either my views or those of my new-age ecofeminist colleagues should define nursing theory."

Mr. J: Which means, if I'm following you correctly, Miss Nightingale, that *both* the explicate and implicate orders have a place in our thinking. Or, to paraphrase the biblical writer: There is a time for everything

MISS N:
under the sun, a time for thinking or acting within the explicate order, and a time for thinking or acting in terms of the implicate order.

MISS N: Yes, thank you, Mr. Jowett. I do appreciate your ability to connect these new ways of thinking to the texts we knew so well in our own time. But let me try to say what this explicate order would be: It would include, as I see it, whatever is mechanistic, highly rational, precisely defined and articulated; that which can be statistically formulated, and studied using a quantitative methodology. And this is *just what we need* for careful prediction, for administrative control, for training young professionals. Also for sorting out our division of labor with fellow professionals (like the "medical men" as I used to call them), and for dealing with politicians.

MR. J: But wait, Miss Nightingale, before you move on to applications of this paradigm, hadn't you better say what you mean by "implicate order?"

MISS N: Of course. By "implicate order" I mean what transcends mechanistic, rational, hierarchical relationships. I mean concepts that serve us best by being allusive, not precise—by serving our explorations instead of our demand for definitions. And I mean orders or patterns that reach beyond our perceptions— that we see, if you like, only "through a glass, darkly." I'm thinking of the order or orders that creative philosophers and poets and painters and musicians reach for. Or the only dimly understood order of wilderness vastness as distinct from the platted settlements; or half-formed new paradigms, as distinct from what they now call normal science. Such orders tend to escape our statistical formulations, and to elude our quantitative methods.

MR. J: This "implicate" order reminds me of that definition of faith in the Epistle to the Hebrews: ". . . the substance of things hoped for, the evidence of things not seen" (Hebrews 11:1). But how, in general, do these explicate and implicate orders relate to one another? Presumably they are not just opposites or contradictories or elements to be balanced off against one another by weight or volume, as on a butcher's scale.

MISS N: Quite. And there's no tidy way to tell when one should leave off thinking of nature as mechanistic and begin relating to it (or Her!?) holistically—as a living organism worthy of reverence. Nor is there a simple rule to tell when my authoritarian way of running a ward should give way to collaborative decision making. But there do seem to be women and men who can make wise judgments about just such matters.

MR. J: And you think, do you, that such wise persons might take the new ecofeminism to be reaching toward the still-unformed implicate order, the larger all-enveloping context, but still recognize the need in some times and places for the rigorous statistical science and forceful administrative leadership you provided as the original foundation for professional nursing?

MISS N: Well, Mr. Jowett, that seems to be where we've got to, isn't it? But perhaps we should get back not to something more specific to nursing theory and practice. You know how I always lost patience with abstract theorizing when I couldn't see its use for solving practical problems.

MR. J: *(smiles)* I do indeed. In fact, I always suspected we'd never have had that 32-year-long correspondence if I had not been an academic administrator besides being a Plato scholar. But tell me about this concept of "the environment." Is it quite important to the way nurses think about their work?

MISS N: It always was for me. But these Boca Raton nurses want to expand the idea to include the whole of nature! And that goes far beyond the individual sick room, or even the public sanitation schemes I used to work on for the military hospitals and, later, for India.

MR. J: Do they suppose that the term "environment" must have only one meaning? Might they not use this explicate–implicate model of David Bohm's that we've been discussing, and think in terms of the islands of immediate environments set in the seas of the less understood, less controllable environment of Nature itself?

MISS N: I think, Mr. Jowett, that would help them to avoid the sorts of false dichotomies we were discussing earlier. But I confess to being a bit unclear myself about how *human agency* fits into their thinking about the nursing environment.

MR. J: *(his brow wrinkling slightly)* Human agency? I'm not sure I understand.

MISS N: Well, as members of a practice discipline and profession, nurses have a special covenant with society to put our knowledge to work—I was always clear in my vision about that responsibility. Putting our knowledge to work is what I mean by agency—being agents of change, specifically of healing. I did this in our day by transforming and creating institutions, like the War Department, the military and civilian hospitals, the workhouses, and public health arrangements. But I thought of myself as separate from the mechanisms of nature, which I had to understand and manipulate to create better environments.

MR. J: I remember all that very well, Miss Nightingale. But I suspect I know what's bothering you. If the ecofeminists urge upon nursing the view of an ultimate implicate order with the character of an all-embracing nurturing organism—Mother Nature, perhaps—you're probably wondering what that means for active manipulation to create health-giving environments.

MISS N: Exactly. On one reading, adopting a vision of the natural environment as a nurturing organism might be seen as encouraging passivity—that we should just let nature take its, or Her, course. From this perspective, *less* human agency, in general, might appear to be an ideal. "Go with the flow" is the phrase I think they sometimes use these days.

MR. J: But they wouldn't have to give up their covenantal responsibility on that view, would they? In *our* time, the belief in a Father–Creator was, for many, the stimulus to serve his will, and, as I believe you said yourself once:

> *God . . . does not treat men like children; mankind is to create mankind. We are to learn, first what* is *heaven, and, secondly, how to* make *it. We are to ascertain what* is *right, and then how to* perform *it. [quoted in Boyd, 1982, p. 215]*

MISS N: I'd never get away among these ecofeminist nurses with talking about "men" and "mankind" like that. But you have a good memory, Mr. Jowett. And your point, I take it, is that interpreting nature as a nurturing home or a nurturing Mother, far from inviting nurses to lean back passively into "the everlasting arms," could be seen as encouragement to be agents themselves of just that sort of nurturing and caring that would put them in harmony with the ultimate meaning of the natural order.

MR. J: Yes, that's what I was getting at. And it connects to what we were saying earlier about how "spirit" and "spirituality" were at the heart of our experience and understanding of our Victorian Christianity, just as they are at the heart of today's ecofeminist thought and practice. But there's one thing more I'd like to hear your thoughts on. Your profession isn't just about environment and human agency—it's essentially about health, is it not? How do your ideas on health fit with what your ecofeminist friends are saying?

MISS N: Well, some of them are saying that we can't nurture the health of our clients if we don't add the health of the whole natural environment to our covenantal responsibility. Some say that human health and environmental health are cocreative of each other. And some call for nurses to become much more political in the service of both human and environmental health—and to do so not just as citizens but as nursing professionals.

MR. J: *(his philosophical mind sensing a conceptual knot to untangle)* Hm . . . But then what's to distinguish a nursing professional from a Green politician, or a Friends of the Earth activist, or an environmental lawyer, or government regulator? Isn't there some risk that, in assigning nurses responsibility for ever-expanding environments—all the way to Nature it-self—the public won't know why they're supporting schools of nursing and nursing instructors won't know what they're to teach?

MISS N: It's a fair point, Mr. Jowett, if not altogether a new one. I wrote in *Notes on Nursing* that *all* women must nurse the sick and prevent illness by working to create clean, light, airy, safe, environments [Nightingale, 1859]. Yet I devoted much of my energy to creating a system of professional education for nurses—with the idea that specialized attention to special health problems was a social need of the highest order. And some would think it paradoxical, I suppose, that I discovered that birthing at home was much safer than the hospital for women and their children, even in poor districts; and yet I spent much effort on creating institutional settings where professional midwifery could be practiced and taught.

MR. J: *(teasing her)* Do I take it, Miss Nightingale, that you *don't know* how professional nurses should take on the health of the whole earth, as it were, as part of their nursing role?

MISS N: Mr. Jowett, would you be putting me on? You do recall how I detest having to say those words, "I don't know."

MR. J: Well . . . ?

MISS N: *(a trifle impatient)* Well, there's something else you will surely remember about me, and that is that I always preferred doing things for sick people to speaking in abstractions. It might not seem so from today's conversation with you, but I once declared my preference "above all other eternities, to work in Hell . . . to save the burning bodies" [quoted in Boyd, 1982, p. 234]. Which reminds me—I must go have a look at the message board outside St. Peter's office. I was promised an answer today to my request to go off on temporary duty to the Lower Regions. I've heard the sanitary conditions there are perfectly horrible. . . . Would you excuse me?

MR. J: My dear Miss Nightingale, how could I possibly say no? You are who you are . . . as am I. . . . Hand me that Greek dictionary, would you?

PERSONAL STATEMENT

As a relatively new philosophy professor, Bob Schultz was prompted to begin teaching courses in environmental ethics when he read Paul Ehrlich's account, in the 1970 *Earth Day Handbook,* of the social and infrastructure implications of 25–30-year population doubling times in some developing countries. That intellectual awakening came together with his love of wilderness to stimulate a commitment that has lasted for over 20 years to offering at least one "environmental" course annually to his liberal arts undergraduates. In 1980, he coedited *Ecological Consciousness: Essays from the Earthday X Colloquium*—the proceedings from a conference of humanities scholars at the University of Denver. From 1983 to 1985, he served as managing editor of *Environmental Review.* Currently, he includes environmental concerns in his work on the policy committee of the Friends Committee on National Legislation, the Quaker lobby in Washington, DC.

Phyllis Schultz's practice and scholarship have centered on the environment in the more specific sense that names the settings where clients become, or remain, healthy, and where nurses organize their delivery of care. She has taught and written in the fields of community health and administration, with particular emphasis on conceptualizing the nature of *client* as more than individual persons. Specifically, she has reasoned that *populations* (or "pluralities of persons") and social interactional entities such as *groups, organizations,* and *communities* are appropriate *nursing clients*—ideas exemplified in Nightingale's earliest writings and in her practice. These extended definitions have necessitated *redefinition* of the other defining concepts in the discipline such as *environment, health,* and *nursing interventions*—conceptualizations of the sort reflected in this chapter. She joins her husband in earth-caring concerns, from recycling in their Brier, Washington, home to sharing values and practical ideas with their grown sons, one an Outward Bound program director, the other a Coast Guard boatswain's mate engaged in fisheries law enforcement and search-and-rescue work.

REFERENCES

Boyd, N. (1982). *Three Victorian women who changed their world.* New York: Oxford University Press.

Cook, Sir Edward. (1913, reissued 1942). *The life of Florence Nightingale.* New York: Macmillan.

May, H. G., & Metzger, B. M. (Eds.). (1962, 1973). *The new Oxford annotated bible.* New York: Oxford University Press.

Merchant, C. (1989). *The death of nature: Women, ecology, and the scientific revolution.* New York: HarperCollins. (With new preface; original work published 1980)

Nightingale, F. (1871). *Introductory notes on lying-in institutions.* London: Longmans, Green.

Nightingale, F. (1859). *Notes on nursing: What it is, and what it is not.* London: Harrison and Sons.

Oelschlaeger, M. (1991). *The idea of wilderness: From prehistory to the age of ecology.* New Haven: Yale University Press.

Quinn, V., & Prest, J. (1987). *Dear Miss Nightingale: A selection of Benjamin Jowett's letters to Florence Nightingale, 1860–1893.* Oxford: Clarendon Press.

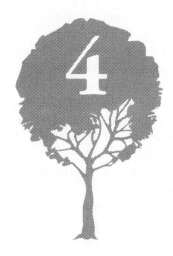

Nurses as Fairies in Gumboots

Bev Taylor

INTRODUCTION

Humans are greater than they know: they are filled with spirit, and this makes them ultimately free. Rather like "fairies in gumboots," humans are interconnected incarnate beings, with bodies of light and love, but with their feet weighted firmly to the ground. Humans are earthed to daily routines and obligations that keep their attention on the apparent emotional polarities of life. In living these routines, they may have forgotten something of their spiritual heritage and their interconnectedness with all things, but, thankfully, their forgetfulness is not complete. The quality of their interpersonal relationships reminds them now and then of the true beauty and power of their human existence.

An awareness of spirit-filled existence has yet to strike the consciousness of many people on earth, but the awareness is growing, and its growth is facilitated to some extent through people-oriented vocations that seek to serve other human beings. Nurses are humans who, by service to others through nursing, have wonderful opportunities to be of use to themselves, to others, and to the planet. Nurses serve humanity through their clinical knowledge and skills, but through their human embodiment they connect all other humans to themselves.

This chapter explores our environmental connections in nursing by focusing on nurses and patients as human beings who are the environment of their own nursing contexts; that is, they are people who relate to one another and to other things by virtue of Being-in-the-world (Gadamer, 1975; Heidegger, 1962) of nursing.

A phenomenological research project describing ordinariness in nursing (Taylor, 1991a) forms the framework of the chapter. That thesis will be extended to suggest some connections between the embodied nature of the nurse–patient relationship and the "magic" that is brought about when sparks of spirit (Capra, 1988; Moore, 1989) unite nurses and patients in their oneness as humans, and with their environment.

Magic happens daily in nursing contexts, even though the fairies in gumboots may not be aware of the full effects of "waving their wands" of love over the people in their care. To the extent that it is possible to know where and when things begin, this chapter starts with the research that sparked my interest in grounding nursing's healing power in the everyday activities of its practitioners.

THE RESEARCH: THE PHENOMENON OF ORDINARINESS IN NURSING

The idea of researching the phenomenon of ordinariness in nursing originated from discussions with Professor Alan Pearson (1988a) about his clinical experiences, and from my own nursing research (Taylor, 1988), in which women expressed a personal preference for the midwives' (who were "just themselves") caring for them.

Essentially, the research used a hermeneutic phenomenological approach to explore the phenomenon of ordinariness in nursing, to illuminate the nature and effect of ordinariness, and to discover whether ordinariness enhances the nursing encounter. Some ideas in phenomenology that informed the theoretical framework of this research were: lived experience (Dilthey, 1985; Gadamer, 1975; Heidegger, 1962; Husserl, 1965, 1970, 1980); Dasein (Heidegger, 1962); Being-in-the-world (Dreyfus, 1991; Heidegger, 1962); and fusion of horizons (Gadamer, 1975).

The nurses, patients, and researcher involved in the research were of various ages and had unique personal histories and circumstances. Each person was regarded as an unique individual, as a Being-in-the-world of the nursing unit, who brought his or her own lived experiences to that context. After I initially distributed a handout and then explained to individuals the aims and processes of the research, six registered nurses, who worked full-time in the Professorial Nursing Unit (PNU), and twenty-four patients in their care consented to participate in the research. The interactions included any nurse–patient communications that were part of the negotiated plan of care for each patient. Informed consent was secured from all the research participants, and the nurses involved informed me when nursing care interactions were scheduled.

The place in which the nurses, patients, and I interacted was a PNU established as a separate nursing area within a traditional hospital organization. People admitted into nursing beds in these units are deemed to require nursing care as their main health need, thus the PNU structures and practices support therapeutic care organized on primary nursing. Nurses in the PNU are allocated periodically to a different team and therefore experience a different mix of leadership style, team composition, and patient case load. Patient care is organized and directed by nurses, and the structure and processes of the units are geared toward making the environment homelike, so that patients can feel as comfortable as possible. Nurses wear street clothes, not uniforms, and patients are encouraged to dress in day clothes and to remain as close as possible to their usual activities of daily living.

Essentially a method of hermeneutical phenomenology, this research used the transcribed text of participants' accounts of their experiences in the world of the PNU to illuminate the phenomenon of ordinariness in nursing. The search for the nature of the phenomenon of ordinariness in nursing began with the context of the people, place, and time and used intersubjective understandings to move toward describing the phenomenon itself.

All of the research participants gave their impressions of the nurse-patient interactions and related areas of interest. After each interaction, I recorded my impressions in my journal, including preinterview and postinterview notes, some demographical information, and a full account of the interaction. As a participant-observer, I interacted with each nurse and patient as appropriate, and I noted the extent and nature of my interactions in my journal as part of my impressions.

After each interaction, a conversation with each patient was audiotaped, in which the only structuring guides were:

I was with you when you interacted with [the nurse] this morning. What did you like about being with [the nurse] this morning? What didn't you like about being with [the nurse] this morning?

It seems likely that what happened was a fairly usual occurrence for [the nurse]. Is there anything about being with [the nurse] that was special for you?

When audiotaping a conversation with each nurse after the respective nurse-patient interactions, the only structuring guide was:

I was with you when you were with [the patient] this morning. Tell me your impressions of being with [the patient] this morning.

The audiotapes were transcribed and, with the journal notes, became text for a hermeneutical interpretation of the respective nurse-patient interactions.

Generating Meaning: The Effects (Qualities and Activities) and Nature (Aspects and Actualities) of Ordinariness in Nursing

As the analysis and interpretation of the participants' impressions unfolded, I found that the phenomenon initially manifested itself by its effects, which, in turn, were reflections of its nature. For the sake of comprehensiveness in the face of brevity, the following account will merge the effects and nature of the phenomenon.

The externalized aspects of the phenomenon of ordinariness in nursing were found to be facilitation, fair play, familiarity, family, favoring, feelings, fun, and friendship, the respective qualities and activities which, in turn, reflected the nature of the phenomenon. These aspects illuminated the phenomenon but did not manifest the nature of the phenomenon itself.

The explication of the nature of ordinariness in nursing had to go beyond the entity (the ontic) to Being (the ontological). A further reimmersion in the text, using the insights already gained, created a new fusion of horizons, which emerged as words that portrayed the "innerness" of each of the aspects: allowingness, straightforwardness, self-likeness, homeliness, favorableness, in-tuneness, lightheartedness, and connectedness. (A fuller account of the methodological rationale for this process is given in Taylor, 1991a.)

Facilitation and Allowingness

Facilitation refers to the enabling qualities and activities of both nurses and patients, whereby certain challenges being experienced by one person are made easier to face by the other person. Some qualities and activities of facilitation include: appreciating skillful nursing care; appreciating help; facilitating independence; facilitating learning; facilitating coping; facilitating comfort; facilitating acceptance of body image changes; facilitating changes; calming fears; building trust; giving confidence; and allowing the experience to unfold.

Allowingness is an actuality of the phenomenon of ordinariness, within which people try to make things easier for other people. In nursing, allowingness creates the potential for patients and nurses to help themselves by providing some guidance and support until such a time, if at all, that people feel able to take over their own daily activities. Allowingness is considerate of the other person's needs to be independent and dignified; it helps quietly and carefully, always attentive to the cues within the other person that suggest a preparedness to resume increasingly autonomous thoughts and actions. Allowingness knows the other for whom it seeks facilitation, because it knows its own enabling nature as part of itself. Allowingness is an actuality of being human; therefore, it recognizes itself in another human and relates to that person through sensitive helping. The nature of allowingness was exemplified beautifully by Sue (nurse) and Becky (patient). Becky said of Sue:

> *I was beginning to think I was just useless, but Sue makes me feel I'm not that bad and I will get better, but it will take time. If I can control the pain. Sue said to me: "If you want me, ring [the buzzer]. When I've wanted her, I've rung and she came and she didn't insist that she help me and that's what I like. She didn't say: "Oh you can't do that. I've got to help you." She just let me go and therefore if I was looking as though I was going to get into trouble she'd help me, but she let me go and let me do it by myself and that's what I want to do . . . I didn't need to be babied, to be told: "Now be careful, don't do this and don't do that!" She just let me go. If I looked as if I was going to get into trouble, she got her hand ready. That's all I wanted. I don't want somebody there, saying: "Careful about this!" Even getting undressed and getting dressed, people said [that] to me. Sue said: "Can you do that? Can you dress and undress yourself?" and I said: "Yes." I know I look awkward doing it, but I've worked out how to do it without hurting myself. Sue just lets me go . . . . I want to try and do things by myself and they just let me go and that's all I want and I feel that I'll get better quicker.*

Fair Play and Straightforwardness

Fair play refers to the sense of reasonableness we possess as humans. Through fair play, we are forthright in saying what we feel we have to say, knowing that the least we can do, even partially, is to tolerate in others frustrating elements that we recognize in ourselves. Some qualities and activities of fair play include straight talking and tolerating one another's humanness.

Straightforwardness is an actuality of the phenomenon of ordinariness, within which people express their thoughts in relation to others. In nursing, straightforwardness creates the potential for patients and nurses to speak to each other as frankly as possible, saying whatever is in need of being said, while at the same time tolerating each other's humanness. Straightforwardness is clear and concise in its delivery and generous in its intent; it speaks to the other to unblock impasses, and it puts the perceived focus of contention plainly on view, to trigger discussion. Straightforwardness knows the other for whom it seeks fair play, because it knows its own nature as part of itself. Straightforwardness is an actuality of being human; therefore, it recognizes itself in another human and relates to that person through sensitive straight-talking.

William (patient) appreciated Peter's (nurse) forthrightness in speaking clearly about what he thought was reasonable. William was making a slow recovery and felt like giving up altogether, but he realized that Peter's straight talk helped him to keep on trying to help himself. William said:

> *He's (Peter has) got his own ideas about things though. As long as he thinks it's doing the job, well, well and good . . . . He's got a sort of "stand over" manner. He thinks he's right and we are all entitled to our opinion. He thinks he's right and he goes ahead and does it. He knows sometimes you don't agree with him. Still, we don't fall out over that . . . . I wouldn't like to see him change his manner . . . . Well, I don't know, in the long run it might help me a lot. I could easily throw my hand in . . . . He reckons it's worth it to keep going. He reckons the results are worth it.*

Familiarity and Self-Likeness

Familiarity refers to that sense we have of someone else, through the sense we have of ourselves, as an individual with a lifetime of experiences. Some qualities and activities of familiarity include: relating to one another's humanness; relating to the other's situation; acknowledging specialness in everyday situations; tolerating noisiness; relating to the patient as person; relating to the nurse as person; relating to each other as people; relating to genuineness in people; equating with a sense of "that's all"; recognizing the days in which everything seems to go wrong; and being part of everyday life.

Self-likeness is an actuality of the phenomenon of ordinariness, within which people see themselves mirrored, to some degree, in other people. In nursing, self-likeness creates the potential for patients and nurses to understand the humanness of themselves in others, to share an affinity as humans who are bonded by the commonality of their ordinary human existence. Self-likeness is the glue of oneness, wherein people share a sense of togetherness, regardless of a vicissitude of differences; it is a source of recognition of Being within human beings, a sense of the ultimate sameness of all people and things in the universe. Self-likeness knows the other for whom it seeks familiarity, because it knows its own human nature as part of itself. Self-likeness is an actuality of being human; therefore, it recognizes itself in another human and connects to that person through sensitive relating.

William (patient) and Peter (nurse) recognized each other as fellow human beings. William talked to Bev (researcher) about how he perceived Peter:

WILLIAM: (I) can't understand how a man like him goes through life not married. (He) comes from around the midlands in England, where my wife came from.

BEV: Oh really! So, you've had a few conversations to him about who he is. Do you think you know him as a person?

WILLIAM: Mm, mm, a fair idea.

BEV: Does that help, do you think?

WILLIAM: Yes. *(starts to cry)* He reminds me a lot of my Queenie.

BEV: He reminds you of someone you know?

WILLIAM: My wife.

BEV: Your wife. She gets onto you and makes you try, does she?

WILLIAM: She's dead now. She had her ideas on life. She was a good woman, a good woman. Yes, he's a bit after her style.

Peter recognized William's present low mental ebb, but he also knew William as a courageous and interesting man.

PETER: He is very down and depressed, and I am not too sure how we are going to get him up again . . . . I think he's [William is] a nice man. When I first met him, he had a great sense of humor, but now he's not quite so lively as he was. He's got a lot of good stories to tell. He went down with the *Canberra* during the war, on the "Archangel" convoys up to Russia. He's got a good few yarns to tell. He's an interesting man.

Family and Homeliness

Family refers to the sense of home we have within ourselves, which binds us to people with whom we have blood ties or special affinities. Some qualities and activities of family include: acknowledging the relevance of family affiliations to the person; expressing familylike ties; appreciating a homelike atmosphere; and preparing to go home.

Homeliness is an actuality of the phenomenon of ordinariness, within which we regard people as family because of either blood ties or special affinities. In nursing, homeliness creates the potential for patients and nurses to develop close interpersonal relationships that encompass perspectives of people as family. Homeliness is sharing common understandings with people and, in so doing, accepting a share of their joys and pains, which are integral to closer human relationships. Homeliness knows the other who is family, because it knows its own bonding nature as part of itself. Homeliness is an actuality of being human; therefore, it recognizes itself in another human and relates to that person through sensitive familylike bonding.

John (patient) was an obese Italian man who had trouble keeping to a diet for diabetes. He was impressed with the amount of freedom he had in the PNU, which allowed him to continue with his usual routines.

> JOHN: Good place . . . . So far, I feel like it at home. Nobody push you around. In the morning, wake up at seven o'clock for insulin. I do it myself. For the last ten years, I can do it.

Elizabeth (nurse) noticed that John enjoyed the homeliness of the PNU.

> ELIZABETH: He seems to have settled in really well and he is treating it like home. He thinks the homely atmosphere is nice. He feels free to come and go as he pleases. He is doing more exercise, which is good. He might continue it when he goes home.

Favoring and 'Favorableness'

Favoring refers to the approval we give to other people and ourselves for commendable qualities that remind us of our essential nature as human beings. Some qualities and activities of favoring include approving commendable human qualities and enjoying statements of appreciation.

Favorableness is an actuality of the phenomenon of ordinariness, within which we are reminded of our own commendable qualities. When we see them in other people, they mirror our essential nature as human beings. In nursing, favorableness creates the potential for patients and nurses to give approval to other people and themselves and, in so doing, to magnify the attractive aspects of themselves and others. Favorableness is seeing beauty in people at the inside level; it recognizes everyday human qualities that defy adequate description, and it realizes that only through sensing them within itself is it able to know that these qualities exist and how they are. Favorableness knows the other for whom it seeks to give favor, because it knows its own pleasing nature as part of itself. Favorableness is an actuality of being human; therefore, it recognizes itself in another human and relates to that person through sensitive favoring.

Ruth (patient) was full of praise for Andrew's (nurse) human qualities.

> RUTH: He doesn't fuss. He's attentive and no fussing. I had a good shower. A lovely shower, and he didn't leave me too long alone. Well he's got such a pleasant personality. A person, a loving, caring person and he is. Yes. He is a loving, caring person.

Andrew enjoyed being around Ruth most of the time, although at times he felt he needed a break from her verbosity.

> ANDREW: Ruth's a good patient to go to when you're feeling down! I don't know. Sometimes with Ruth you feel like saying, "Oh, please Ruth, just shut up!" But I mean she's nice and bright.

Feelings and In-Tuneness

Feelings are the way we sense ourselves in relation to our worlds of people and things: sometimes as feeling high, sometimes as feeling low, sometimes as feeling somewhere in between. Some qualities and activities of feelings include acknowledging the polarity of human feelings and expressing feelings.

In-tuneness is an actuality of the phenomenon of ordinariness, within which we are sensitive to our feelings and express them as a legitimate part of ourselves and the polarity of things within our worlds. In nursing, in-tuneness creates the potential for patients and nurses to acknowledge and express, to themselves and one another, the polarity of their feelings. In-tuneness is clearing away the debris of rationality in order to face up to, and embrace, the rawness of emotions. Expression of emotions unblocks the streams of human reactivity and causes our life energies to flow a little easier. In-tuneness knows the other with whom it seeks to share its feelings, because it knows its own feeling nature as part of itself. In-tuneness is an actuality of being human; therefore, it recognizes itself in another human and relates to that person through sensitive expressions of feeling.

Jane (nurse) expressed how she felt in relation to being the one to discuss with Max (patient, with triplegia) whether he wished to be resuscitated, should his heart stop beating. Jane said:

> *I don't know. I've said basically a lot of my nursing is gut feeling. I can't explain, but I think I'll know [when the time comes to discuss resuscitation with Max] . . . . I think it will feel bloody awful. I'm not looking forward to it one little bit . . . . Personally, myself, I would like that choice [of whether or not I wanted to be resuscitated] . . . . But I'm just thinking of Max as a person, as a patient being poked at, or whatever label you want to put on it. I just think that he has that right [to decide for himself].*

Fun and Lightheartedness

Fun refers to a sense of merriment that lightens our day-to-day lives and reacquaints us with the child within us all. Some qualities and activities of fun include enjoying a sense of humor.

Lightheartedness is an actuality of the phenomenon of ordinariness, within which we share our sense of fun. In nursing, lightheartedness creates the potential for patients and nurses to express themselves through the medium of humor. Lightheartedness is levity above the everyday circumstances that cloud our minds and weigh our bodies down. Lightheartedness seeks to aerate the lead ball of life and turn it into a bright balloon. Lightheartedness knows the other for whom it seeks humor, because it knows its own laughing nature as part of itself. Lightheartedness is an actuality of being human; therefore, it recognizes itself in another human and relates to that person through sensitive humoring.

Ralph (patient) teased Sue (nurse) about the length of her fingernails, prior to her giving him a back massage.

RALPH: So I said to Sue, whose nails weren't all that short before she started: "Let's have a look at your nails," jokingly, because she's five stone heavier than me! So she jokingly said: "They're alright." With that over, we proceeded. So she said: "He's been reading up, he's checking on me." Oh no, [I was] quite at ease. I was looking forward to it. That's why I thought I'd better read up a bit on this massage business, just so I could sling off and try and find something wrong with the deal on the way through, but I couldn't.

Ralph joked about Sue's size, but he was quick to correct any misconception his humor may have caused.

RALPH: Meaning, she could have a bit of German in her. I reckon she could punch like a tank—not that she'd ever do that, of course. You couldn't faze her. I've seen her here with some fairly obnoxious sort of people and she has them laughing within two minutes. Oh no, she could handle all situations. Yeah, she's good.

Friendship and Connectedness

Friendship refers to knowing people well enough to regard them with affection. Some qualities and activities of friendship include: acknowledging the importance of company and talking; expressing affection and liking; and taking time to know one another.

Connectedness is an actuality of the phenomenon of ordinariness, within which we sense ourselves as friends. In nursing, connectedness creates the potential for patients and nurses to know one another well enough to regard each other with affection. Connectedness is recognizing friendly aspects in other people and coming in closer to get to know them. Connectedness takes time; people get to know each other person through keeping company and talking. Connectedness knows the other with whom it seeks friendship, because it knows its own befriending nature as part of itself. Connectedness is an actuality of being human; therefore, it recognizes itself in another human and relates to that person through sensitive liking.

The nature of connectedness is exemplified well by the relationship among Sally (nurse), Sophie (nurse), and Gus (patient). Following the amputation of one of his legs, Gus suffered phantom pain, especially at night. He survived the early morning hours, knowing that Sally and Sophie were there to be with him. Gus acknowledged the importance of company and talk.

> *Well, myself, I found it [the conversation with Sally] good. I mean to say, she's a busy girl and I could talk to her all day and all night. Do you know what I mean? Well, they'll [the nurses will] do anything for you, to help you. Anytime. I could sit here all night and I'd still get my cups of tea or coffee and all that. They'd come in at nighttime, 'cause I'd be in trouble at nighttime. I used to prop that [the amputated leg] and make a noise some nights. They'd hear me, and they'd come in and say: "I don't think that this [the phantom pain] can be fixed. It's gotta just take its own course, I think."*

Sally acknowledged the importance of being with Gus during the night.

> SALLY: It was just a bit of a chat, because there's not a lot that we actually do physically or whatever with him at night. So, it's to let him know that we have time for him, even though we are not necessarily doing a task.

To reiterate the introduction to this section, the externalized aspects of the phenomenon of ordinariness in nursing were found to be facilitation, fair play, familiarity, family, favoring, feelings, fun, and friendship, the respective qualities and activities of which were the effects of the phenomenon. It was recognized that these aspects illuminated the phenomenon, but that they did not manifest the nature of the phenomenon itself. To explicate the nature of ordinariness in nursing, I went beyond the ontic to the ontological, in order to describe the "innerness" of each of the aspects. I found that: within facilitation there is allowingness; within fair play there is straightforwardness; within familiarity there is self-likeness; within family there is homeliness; within favoring there is favorableness; within feelings there is in-tuneness, within fun there is lightheartedness, and within friendship there is connectedness.

SOME POSSIBILITIES FOR NURSING PRACTICE

Nurses involved in day-to-day practice interact more frequently and intimately with patients than any other health professionals; therefore, they may find possibilities for enhancing the therapeutic value of their practice by attending to the meanings generated in this research. As the hub of nursing, the nurse–patient relationship is at the heart of what matters in nursing (Pearson, 1988b). Nurses who feel an affinity with these meanings and deem them to be appropriate for enhancing their own practice of nursing, may use each of the aspects (and their respective actualities) to increase the quality of their nurse–patient relationships, thus potentiating their therapeutic effects.

SUMMARY

The phenomenological research for this chapter found that nurses and patients shared a common sense of humanity, which enhanced the nurse–patient encounter. Within the context of caring, the nurses were ordinary people perceived as being extraordinarily effective because of the ways in which their humanness shone through their knowledge and skills, making their whole being with patients something more than just professional helping.

The patients attuned themselves with the nurses because of their sense of affinity with the nurses as humans. At the same time, the patients acknowledged the nurses' knowledge and skills and allowed themselves to be supported by the nurses' professional qualities and activities. The shared sense of ordinariness between nurses and patients made them as one in their humanness and created a special place in which the relative strangeness of the experience of being in a health care setting could be made familiar and manageable.

BEYOND ORDINARINESS IN NURSING

In exploring our environmental connections in nursing, we need to focus on nurses and patients as human beings, because they are the environment of their own nursing contexts. They are people who relate to one another and to other things in their worlds; thus, they are, at once, part of the whole by virtue of Being-in-the-world (Gadamer, 1975; Heidegger, 1962) of nursing.

The work of clinical nursing contributes to therapeutic patient outcomes and attests to the value of nurses and patients "being themselves" as human beings, in the relatively strange context of the health care setting. Nurses' and patients' connectedness as humans transcends any professional differences they might have, and unifies them in the nurse–patient relationship, so that the ordinariness of being human, defined as a sense of shared humanity (Taylor, 1991a, 1991b, 1992a, 1992b), becomes a powerful source of connectedness and healing. It is as though nurses and patients recognize one another as humans through a sensing that acknowledges, albeit implicitly, that they are spirit-filled beings, earthed in their "gumboots" of humanity by their allowingness, straightforwardness, self-likeness, homeliness, favorableness, intuneness, lightheartedness, and connectedness (Taylor, 1991a).

Nurses Claiming Their Human Potential: From Helpers to Human and Healers

As a practice discipline, nursing has struggled to explicate the nature of its work and the effects that its practice has on people. I have argued elsewhere (Taylor, 1992a, 1992b) that many of the descriptions portraying nurses solely as professional helpers have robbed them of some of their inherent humanness, and, thereby, have disconnected them from the very source of their human potential of caring and healing. Regardless of their professional role relationships and functions, nurse–patient relationships remain essentially human, embodying all the fundamentally ordinary qualities of people interacting in their worlds.

The claim has been made that care is the essence of nursing (Leininger, 1985; Watson, 1985) and that nursing is both carative and curative (Benner & Wrubel, 1989; Kitson, 1984; Pearson, 1988c). The word *therapeutic* is derived from the Greek *therapeutikos,* meaning to nurse, serve, or cure (Webster, 1971). Defined thus, the healing potential of therapeutic nursing is related to the science of nursing, as well as to the artistry with which nursing care is given.

Peplau (1952) first introduced into the literature a description of nursing as a therapeutic relationship. Nurse-scholars (McMahon & Pearson, 1991; Pearson, 1988c, 1988d) are beginning to explore the therapeutic potential of nursing, in terms of its healing possibilities. Claims for therapeutic effects in nursing have arisen from authors' interpretations of the nature of the nurse-patient relationship. Pearson (1988c, p. 12) claimed that exploration of therapeutic approaches in nursing care "can get at the heart of practice," that is, into the nurse-patient relationship, when professional detachment is abandoned in favor of "closeness between nurse and patient, the idea of partnership, and the development of empathy in nursing." The effect of this closeness is considered to be healing in nature, so that nursing care is regarded as therapy (McMahon & Pearson, 1991).

The therapeutic nature of nursing is related to the healing effects of nurses and patients interacting as humans together. Something more than nurses' knowledge and skills accounts for the healing effects, because the therapeutic effects are reciprocated between nurses and patients. Therapeutic nursing is related to the quality of the nurse-patient relationship and how this relationship mobilizes healing responses in individuals. Therefore, valuing therapeutic nursing is the same as valuing the nurse-patient relationship as a potentiating force in health care.

SEARCHING FOR THE SOURCE OF THERAPEUTIC NURSING

The nature of caring and curing in nursing has been explicated to some extent, but, to date, no actual energizing and enabling source of therapeutic nursing has been suggested, other than the nature of human interaction itself. It is the bold assertion of this chapter that nurses will know intuitively the source of the healing that comes through therapeutic nursing. Healing, as you well know, is not necessarily slicing, dicing, testing, and ingesting; healing is caring, loving, accepting, and knowing with the inner heart in service to all. Healing is a human potential. To heal with the inner heart is simply a matter of "returning home" to remember and recognize the essence of one's humanness. Returning home is listening to the inner voice of knowing, that knowing that hears the scholarly arguments of the empirico-analytical world, and says: "Yes, but . . . ."

The Path Homeward

For some people like McFerrin (1988), the path homeward to the spirit within is one they take without further ado; for others like Capra (1988), it is a matter of finding it through some form of rationality.

In the foreword of his little book entitled *Don't Worry, Be Happy,* Bobby McFerrin (1988) wrote these profoundly simple words:

> *I believe that life is fundamentally benevolent and people are basically good and know what's good for them. Things have a way of righting themselves without much meddling. No matter what those things are, big things, middle things, little things, I know we are bigger and greater than anything we meet along the way and we instinctively confront, bear down on and conquer anything that ails the collective soul. I know I'm part of everything. I'm part of nature and I know nature doesn't worry.*

In his book, *Uncommon Wisdom: Conversations with Remarkable People,* Fritjof Capra (1988) recorded a discussion he enjoyed with R. D. Laing about two seemingly different views of consciousness. They agreed that the Western scientific view of consciousness considers matter as primary, and consciousness as a property of complex material patterns that emerge by a process of biological evolution. The other main view is what may be called the mystical view: consciousness is the primary reality, the essence of the universe, the ground of all Being; and everything else—all forms of matter and living beings—are manifestations of pure consciousness. This view is based on nonordinary modes of awareness, and as such it is regarded as indescribable.

When they considered an example of natural beauty, however, such as the place in which they stood as the sunset settled over the ocean, Capra and Laing agreed that its sights, sounds, and smells were indescribable, and that not only mystical experiences, but also "any experience of reality is indescribable" (Capra, 1988, p. 142), because humans can take in the context of a single moment, yet they are not able to describe fully that experience.

They proceeded to connect rationally the two seemingly different views of human consciousness.

> *The systems view of life agrees with the traditional scientific view, that consciousness is a property of complex material patterns, [precisely] a property of living things at a certain complexity. On the other hand, the biological structures of these systems are manifestations of underlying processes, . . . the process of self-organisation, . . . identified as mental processes. In this sense, biological processes are manifestations of mind . . . . [Extended] . . . to the universe as a whole, [it could be said] that all of its structures—from subatomic particles to galaxies and from bacteria to human beings—are manifestations of the universal dynamics of self-organisation, which means the cosmic mind. And this, more or less the mystical view. (p. 143)*

Thus, Capra and Laing argued that the systems view of life can provide a meaningful framework for connecting the traditional approaches to questions of life, mind and consciousness, and those put forward by the so-called mystical views. To get back to the original reason for this digression, McFerrin, Capra, and Laing have a sense of the connectedness of human consciousness, through their own ways of knowing. People may find a path homeward to the energizing source of their humanness through a variety of means, such as the sacred writings (The Bhagavadgita, 1962; The Koran, 1974; The New English Bible, 1971), writings that are compilations of religious traditions (Hughes, 1942; Rhys Davids, 1956–1966; Waley, 1958), so called "new age" publications (Houston, 1990; Malone & Malone, 1987; Millman, 1992; Moore, 1989) and, of course, the personal instruction that comes from the experience of one's own life lessons. You will know which is the best way for you.

THE FUTURE FOR FAIRIES IN GUMBOOTS

What is the future for fairies in gumboots, especially those who choose to be of service to others through nursing practice? Like all other humans, nurses are actually quite extraordinary. Nurses are special in their uniqueness, a phenomenon often forgotten, or taken for granted, in the familiarity of everyday embodied existence. Although some nurses use actively in nursing their holistic perceptions and practices (Kreiger, 1985, in Kunz, 1985), a widespread acceptance or acknowledgment of nurses' humanness and of the inherent spiritual essence of humanity is not apparent.

This chapter has used the metaphor of fairies in gumboots, and even though Gardner (1982) might argue that these spirit-filled beings do, in fact, exist, this has not been a contention here. The metaphor was used to convey the meaning that, as fairies in gumboots, humans are interconnected incarnate beings who have their feet weighted firmly to the ground. Humans are earthed to daily routines and obligations that keep their attention focused on the apparent emotional polarities of life. What has been suggested is that humans are greater than they know. Humans are spirit-filled beings of love and light and, as such, they are a part of all there is. When we, as humans, gain a sense of this oneness, we need never feel small, insignificant, and lonely again. Because humans are gaining a firmer and firmer sense of their spiritual heritage, the future looks bright for all people and for the healing of the planet. In our particular interests, the future looks bright for nurses as fairies in gumboots and for the work they do in their daily practice.

CONCLUSION

This chapter has suggested that humans are greater than they know. Because they are filled with spirit, they are ultimately free. They may have forgotten something of their spiritual heritage and their interconnectedness with all things, but their forgetfulness is not complete. The quality of their interpersonal relationships reminds them now and then of the true beauty and power of their human existence.

Through their service to others, nurses have wonderful opportunities to be of use to themselves, to others, and to the planet. The nurse–patient relationship is a source of healing when nurses and patients allow the love of their human interconnectedness to become a form of therapy. A phenomenological research project describing the phenomenon of ordinariness in nursing (Taylor, 1991a) formed the framework of this chapter, and it was the starting point for an extension of that thesis. This natural extension of ordinariness in nursing reiterates an old awareness and puts it into a new context. Simply stated: there are interconnections among all people, and in the embodied nature of the nurse–patient relationship, the magic that is brought about by those sparks of spirit (Capra, 1988; Moore, 1989) unites nurses and patients as one with each other and with their environment. In this sense, we are all one with all there is; there is no separation.

PERSONAL STATEMENT

I have interpreted the theme of environment in the sense of the individual as a spiritual being within the broader context of physical and social relations. Within this idea is the notion that human beings are people whose bodies are the environment for their own spirits, and, collectively, they form groups of people who relate to the broader environment of the planet. The integrity of an individual's personal environment, therefore, relates to the ultimate integrity of the planet, in that the vibrations generated by the daily spiritual walk of the person affect the collective vibration of the earth as it seeks to heal itself. Therefore, my interpretation of environment in this chapter is in relation to the internal spiritual environment of people and how this in turn affects, and is affected by, the broader context of the earth as environment.

REFERENCES

Benner, P., & Wrubel, J. (1989). *The primacy of caring: Stress and coping in health and illness.* Menlo Park, CA: Addison-Wesley.

Capra, F. (1988). *Uncommon wisdom: Conversations with remarkable people.* London: Fontana Paperbacks.

Dilthey, W. (1985). *Poetry and experience. Selected works* (Vol. V). Princeton, NJ: Princeton University Press.

Dreyfus, H. L. (1991). *Being-in-the-world:* A commentary on Heidegger's being and time, division 1. Cambridge, MA: MIT Press.

Gadamer, H. G. (1975). *Truth and method.* G. Barden (Ed.) & J. Cumming (Trans.). Seabury, NY.

Gardner, L. E. (1982). *Pictures of fairies: The Cottingley photographs.* First Quest Edition. Wheaton, IL: Theosophical Publishing House.

Heidegger, M. (1962). *Being and time.* J. Macquarrie & E. Robinson (Trans.). New York: Harper & Row.

Houston, J. (1990). *The search for the beloved: Journeys in sacred psychology.* Los Angeles, CA: J. P. Tharcher.

Hughes, E. R. (1942). *The great learning and the meaning-in-action.* (Newly translated from the Chinese, with an introductory essay on the history of Chinese philosophy.) London: J. M. Dent.

Husserl, E. (1965). *Phenomenology and the crisis of philosophy.* Q. Lauer (Trans.). New York: Harper & Row.

Husserl, E. (1970). *The crisis of the European sciences and transcendental phenomenology.* Evanston, IL: Northwestern University Press.

Husserl, E. (1980). *Phenomenology and the foundations of the sciences.* T. E. Klein & W. E. Pohl (Trans.). The Hague: Martinus Nijhoff.

Kitson, A. L. (1984). *Steps towards the identification and development of nursing therapeutic functions in the care of hospitalised elderly.* Unpublished doctoral dissertation, University of Ulster, Coleraine.

Kunz, D. (1985). *Spiritual aspects of the healing arts.* Wheaton, IL: Theosophical Publishing House.

Leininger, M. (1985). *Qualitative research methods in nursing.* New York: Grune & Stratton.

Malone, T. P., & Malone, P. T. (1987). *The art of intimacy.* Englewood Cliffs, NJ: Prentice-Hall.

McFerrin, B. (1988). *Don't worry, be happy.* New York: Delacorte Press.

McMahon, R., & Pearson, A. (Eds.). (1991). *Nursing as therapy.* London: Chapman and Hall.

Millman, D. (1992). *No ordinary moments: A peaceful warrior's guide to daily life.* Tiburon, CA: H. J. Kramer.

Moore, M. M. (1989). *Bartholomew: Reflections of an elder brother.* Taos, NM: High Mesa Press.

Pearson, A. (1988a). *Just an ordinary nurse.* Lakeside Graduation Address (unpublished).

Pearson, A. (Ed.). (1988b). *Primary nursing.* London: Croom Helm.

Pearson, A. (1988c). *Therapeutic nursing—The effects of admission to a nursing unit.* Oxford, England: Oxfordshire Health Authority.

Pearson, A. (1988d, August). *Therapeutic nursing: The effect of admission to a nursing unit on patient outcome.* Paper presented to Future Directions Conference, SA Health Commission, Adelaide, Australia.

Peplau, H. E. (1952). *Interpersonal relations in nursing.* New York: Putnam.

Rhys Davids, T. W. (1956–1966). Dialogue of the Buddha, in *Sacred books of the Buddhists,* Translated from the Pali. London: Luzac.

Taylor, B. J. (1988). *What are the patients' perceptions of the usefulness of information given to them by nurses and what are the nurses' perceptions of their roles and constraints as teachers in giving effective patient education in a postnatal ward?* Research paper submitted in partial fulfillment of the requirements for the degree of Master of Education, Deakin University, Geelong, Australia.

Taylor, B. J. (1991a). *The phenomenon of ordinariness in nursing.* Unpublished doctoral dissertation, Deakin University, Geelong, Australia.

Taylor, B. J. (1991b). *The dialectic of the nurse as person: Ordinary nurses perceived as extraordinarily effective.* Proceedings, Conference on Science, Reflectivity and Nursing Care: Exploring the Dialectic, Melbourne, Australia.

Taylor, B. J. (1992a). Relieving pain through ordinariness in nursing: A phenomenological account of a comforting nurse–patient encounter. *Advances in Nursing Science,* Vol. I, pp. 33–43.

Taylor, B. J. (1992b). From helper to human: A reconceptualisation of the nurse as person. *Journal of Advanced Nursing, 17,* 1042–1049.

The Bhagavadgita. (1962). Translated from the Sanskrit with an introduction by Juan Mascaro. Baltimore: Penguin Books.

The Koran. (1974). Translated from the Arabic with notes by N. J. Dawood (4th ed.). Hammondsworth, England: Penguin.

The New English Bible. (1971). New York: Cambridge University Press.

Waley, A. (1958). *The way and its power: A study of the Tao te Ching and its place in Chinese thought.* New York: Grove Press.

Watson, J. (1985). *Nursing: Human science and human care. A theory of nursing.* Norwalk, CT: Appleton-Century-Crofts.

Webster, N. (1971). The International Webster Encyclopedic Dictionary. New York: Tabor House.

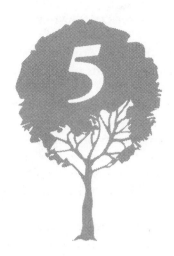

Exploring Ethical Ways of Being with Another and Earth, Including Life-Style Changes to Promote a Culture of Simplicity

Joyce C. Kadandara

As nurses across frontiers, we are aware that the right to health is the most basic of all human rights. Every human being, even in the remotest part of Africa, has the right to live in an environment with minimum risks. We know many of the Earth's people are now being adversely affected by the physical environment in which they live. For example, ozone-depleting gases from manufacturing processes have been found to cause health problems.

The challenges facing the health sector before the year 2000 in Zimbabwe, as in other African nations, are formidable. The nursing profession must address, in the most serious manner, all environmental issues that affect the quality of life of many of our people. The changes in weather patterns, which have confused my 100-year-old grandmother, have also adversely affected our harvests and increased the levels of malnutrition in our children, our women, and our aged.

Our lives depend largely on agricultural outputs. They are the major source of income for many people. Deny them a good harvest because of changes in the weather patterns, and they face an "epidemic of poverty." The world media have brought into your homes the suffering experienced by many people in a variety of settings, mostly in the developing nations. A variety of causes have been identified: socioeconomic reasons, political reasons, climatic reasons, lack of education, lack of skills to generate new industries, and so on.

Whatever the reasons we might want to put forward, the questions that we, as a caring profession, need to ask are:

How have nations, both developed and underdeveloped, allowed such a sorry state of affairs to occur and expand?

What have we, as health professionals, done?

Is it not our role to be advocates of our communities in health issues?

Women and children around the world presently suffer from the most debilitating diseases know to humanity. These ailments include chronic anemia, malnutrition, and severe fatigue. They all stem from poor food intake and women's excessive work loads, and they are all preventable. This is the irony of this problem.

As nurses, we must begin to push the boundaries of our peoples' health beyond disease patterns and classifications to encompass the entire life cycle and to include key nonmedical factors, such as the environment, that have profound influence on the well-being of individuals, families, and communities. They should have a quality of life, not mere existence. Quality assurance in the health care system will only be meaningful when the world's marginalized people begin to be cared for according to their needs.

The world we live in is not a fair one. We have seen social, economic, and political disturbances, and deadly wars, in many areas of the globe. The factors causing these unrests could have been prevented if the world we live in had been prepared to accommodate varying viewpoints.

We cannot expect to live in a world of peace and tranquillity if governments do not agree on an agenda for change. Health and environmental issues are secondary to guns being bought or supplied. Very few people have any compassion for the poverty-ridden masses of the world or even for those in their own backyards. There are no set standards of how countries should behave in their quest to better themselves and amass more wealth. The focus is on buying more weapons that destroy people not on the health care needed to save them.

Weapons of destruction are not only guns and ammunition. They are also the industrial emissions of unacceptable levels of chlorofluorocarbons (CFCs), which cause depletion in the ozone layer and, in turn, destroy the environment we live in. There is no universal code of ethics among the nations on how we should manage our beautiful Earth. The international conference on the environment in 1992 brought home to us the division that continues between the haves and the have nots. The have nots in my part of the world, Africa, are in the majority and their lot is dictated by those who have made it in life.

Some of the research on the environment reveals serious exposure of the world's population to health hazards, both in homes and in industries. The burning of biomass fuels used in cooking and heating inside homes, the carrying of heavy loads of water and firewood, and similar daily tasks in various cultures, have a negative effect on individuals' health. Proximity to household stoves has been linked to increased prevalence of chronic bronchitis (Chen et al., 1990).

In most parts of the world, women spend more time than men cooking indoors, and therefore are at higher risk. When we look back on the history of my country, it is evident that our people lived a simple life that was in unison with the environment. We had our own problems and our endemic disease patterns, but on the whole our forests were lush and green, the fruits of the wild were plentiful, and the wild animals that roamed our forests provided the communities with nutritious meat to eat. In 1890, when my country, Zimbabwe, was colonized, "all hell broke loose." There was a change in our life-styles, our disease patterns, and our culture.

Our rural folk were moved from fertile grounds free from diseases to poor and unproductive areas that are rich in mosquitoes. The diseases they contracted brought suffering to many people, and many died. Today, we are struggling to eliminate poverty and to prevent diseases. The natural resources we could now be using much more effectively, have long been carried away from the country or have been exhausted. The struggle has not been and will not be easy.

The environmental degradation has also been caused by the need for shelter, warmth, and food. Natural trees have been cut to build homes and provide fuel for many rural folk. This results in soil erosion and poor crop yields.

Diseases caused by contaminated water supplies and lack of proper sanitation could have been minimized or completely eliminated if only a small percentage of the plundered wealth realized by our colonizers had been earmarked for rural development. Ninety years of neglect are now being addressed. We gained our independence in 1980. We still have a long way to catch up.

Many environmental factors have a major bearing on mothers and children, who, by the very nature of our societies, suffer discrimination. Day by day, they become more and more vulnerable. Women have been identified as the foremost providers of primary health care. They are also the producers of mankind. Unless we take care of this endangered species, there won't be any mankind—or womankind, for that matter—left in this world.

Many of our people know about the changes in the weather patterns. They wonder why the Almighty is punishing them. What they do not know about are the ozone-layer changes that scientists have identified. The world's major environmental problems are not caused by the poor people of Africa; they are caused by those who have a better life and have, in the past, caused environmental degradation with impunity. Why should the developed world care about the people in far-off places, like rural Africa? Is it not human to love thy world neighbor as thyself? We need to *be* one another; we need to care. We need a code of international ethics that dictates how we should behave on issues that affect all of us. We need to promote a culture of simplicity for all, especially those in the developed world. We have a culture of simplicity in Africa. We cannot get any simpler, otherwise we will cease to exist.

We acknowledge that modern life is here to stay. We are helping in analyzing positive ways of being with one another and with Earth. The environment is our tree of life. Let us nurture it with love, care, and understanding. We need to act locally and think globally on all environmental issues. Modern technology has brought many positive advances, but some of the technology has negative end-results that have not been sensitive to the particular health needs of many of our people, especially our women and children. The use of heavy machinery, which is cumbersome and emits smoke or exhaust, has caused harm to many people. We need to find other means of supporting the environment. Alternative sources of energy are needed in many parts of Africa. Good sanitary facilities, adequate food and clean water supplies, and acceptable homes are prerequisites to health. However, because of poverty, many of our people still do not have these basic health needs. We have worked hard for very little. We need to feel we are equal partners in dealing with environmental issues.

The developed countries have industrialized and should assign themselves a bigger role in the reduction of CFCs. The developing world will also play its role, but development of its industries has also to take place.

Many of our governments signed the documents on the environment in Rio de Janeiro, but some member states were not prepared to do so because the standard of living of their people would be affected. What will happen to our beautiful Earth if we all take the same uncompromising stance?

The developing world needs the basic things in life. We need to maintain our culture and our simple lives. However, we cannot be the only ones to sacrifice our lives when others are abusing the environment with increased emissions from industries, without a second thought.

Nursing has a role to play in delivering good health. It must also play an effective role in influencing policies related to health and human suffering. The good basics in life, like food, shelter, clean water, and proper sanitation, are some of the goals we in our part of the world are trying to achieve. We need to move some of our advocacy out of the hospital wards and start being heard more in committees that are dealing with environmental issues.

Nobody likes to come into this world poor *and* die poor. For most people in the developing world, the reality of being born poor and dying poor is always there. Life is a right to all of us. As "specialists of life," let us protect the environment, which is our tree of life. Nurses should face the environmental challenge together and put nursing in the forefront of exploring ethical ways of being with one another and Earth.

Our life-styles have to change, but change should be for all of us, not only the people of the developing world.

The world is one; therefore, its people should live as one.

PERSONAL STATEMENT

I grew up in the beautiful country of Zimbabwe, in the southern part of Africa. My country's population of 10.4 million includes all races, but the majority is composed of the indigenous African whose history and culture date back many centuries. I was born in rural Zimbabwe. The birds of the wild woke me every morning to a clear sky and the red Sun rising in the horizon. The morning dew watered the grass, the trees, and the beautiful, scented flowers. My feet were bathed in the dew as I started running to school every morning on a gravel path.

There were no cars to pollute the air and endanger life. The countryside was a haven of peace. I am the firstborn of a family of eight children, six girls and two boys. My parents gave me the love and care that make me appreciate the joy of family unity and support. I was a bright student and an award winner right through my junior and high schools.

I was interested in caring for the sick and disadvantaged members of my community from an early age. I therefore entered a nursing school in Zimbabwe. When I left in my second year and went to England, I had to start nursing all over again. I completed training in 1965. I am a trained nurse and midwife and an experienced ophthalmic theater sister. I am now a widow with two grown sons. I began university studies as a mature student, and graduated with an honors degree in sociology and public administration. I also earned a postgraduate diploma in social administration. My academic qualifications and training were obtained in Rhodesia (now Zimbabwe) and the United Kingdom.

I have invested over thirty-five years of my life in caring for the sick and disadvantaged. Poverty still affects many of my people, but Zimbabweans are a determined and proud nation who fought for their independence and are now fighting to break the chains of deprivation.

I enjoy the good things that nature provides. I am concerned about the degradation of the environment and try to maintain the natural vegetation around my home and encourage my neighbors to do the same. My country cannot escape the need to industrialize. I hope that, as the acceleration for industrial "takeoff" occurs, my children, my grandchildren, and all Zimbabweans will be aware of the growing danger from the ozone layer's depletion.

I still walk barefoot in my garden, and the morning dew bathes my feet and reminds me of the joys of being healthy and alive, and of breathing clean, fresh air touched with the scent of flowers. The clear sky and moonlit nights make me happy to belong to this beautiful country of Zimbabwe, a resident of the beautiful continent called Africa.

REFERENCES

Chen, B. H., et al. (1990). Indoor pollution in developing countries. *World Health Statistics Quarterly, 43*(3), 127–138.

Ministry of Health, Zimbabwe. (1984). *Equity in health.* Ministry of Health Publication.

Ministry of Health, Zimbabwe/UNICEF. (1985). Children and women in Zimbabwe. A situational analysis. Ministry of Health/UNICEF Publication.

United Nations. (1991). *Women: Challenges to the year 2000.* New York: United Nations.

Women's health at the crossroads: Excerpts from the health of women: A global perspective. (1993). M. A. Koblinsky, J. Timyan, & J. Gay (Eds.). Boulder, CO: Westview Press.

Women's health: Across age and frontier. (1992). Geneva: World Health Organization.

World Health Organization. (1988). *Leadership in health:* WHO Forum 9. Geneva, Switzerland.

Zimbabwe Service Availability Survey. (1989/1990). Central Statistical Office, Ministry of Finance, Economic Planning, and Development, Harare, Zimbabwe. Available from Demographic and Health Surveys Institute for Resource Development/Macro International Inc., Columbia, MD.

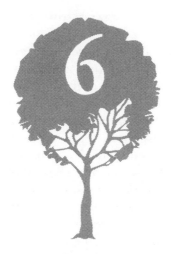

The Bright Alps Project: Creating Caring Environments for People with Disabilities

Susan Elsom

When we talk about nursing and the environment, we often get distracted by the more immediate and very visible problems of throwaway plastics, single-use-only equipment, and the massive "waste creation bias" of the health industry. Although these problems are far from being trivial, they often hide the more intangible and more dehumanizing processes that accompany environmental abuse.

Our blatant and most wasteful abuse of the physical environment reflects the disharmony within ourselves—a disharmony fed by attitudes of irreverence, disrespectfulness, hostility, intolerance, and extreme arrogance. Our arrogance feeds the illusion that humans are made to conquer and control creation rather than be a part of it. Not only do humans attempt to control and overpower the environment, they also engage in a more devious and often subconscious abuse of the human spirit. This "rape" of the human spirit ultimately generates intense feelings of despair and anxiety, an overwhelming sense of powerlessness, and, finally, a pitiful acquiescence.

Nowhere has this been more clearly demonstrated than within the deprived and neglected environment of the mental retardation institutions where I worked for several years. Because I trained and practiced my nursing inside its walls, and because I, like the people for whom I cared, became part of the dehumanizing processes typifying institutional environments, I feel a great necessity to write about some of my experiences and to warn others of the chaos and disharmony that result from a lack of caring for the human spirit.

Wolf Wolfensberger (1972), a well-known advocate for people with disabilities and a critic of institutional life, describes an "institution" as:

> *[a] deindividualising residence in which persons are congregated in numbers distinctly larger than might be found in a large family; in which they are highly regimented; in which the physical and social environment aims at the lowest common denominator; in which all transactions of daily life are carried on under the roof, on one campus, or in a largely segregated fashion. (p. v)*

In 1985, Wolfensberger went on to emphasize the "low value" placed on those inside institutions and made a most chilling observation: these "devalued persons almost certainly will be badly treated."

Wolfensberger's description presents a powerful enough image of mental retardation institutions, but I would posit that it could very aptly be applied to our institutionalized world of today. With our sophisticated bureaucracies and technocracies, our economic rationalists and "user pays" systems, the world in which we live may well be described as "a deindividualizing residence."

I believe that the very foundations of institutions that house intellectually and physically disabled people were built on the premise that these people were deviant and irredeemable social misfits who manifested unacceptable behaviors that threatened normal social functioning. They were perceived as abominations of creation, not integral parts of it.

The hard brick walls, the cold concrete floors, and the spartan style dormitories epitomized the social attitudes of the day and set the scene for harsh and restrictive care practices that depersonalized the patients and destroyed their sense of humanness. Citizens living "outside" remained blissfully oblivious to the dehumanizing processes within, and preferred to believe that deviance was a product of inheritance rather than of socialization. The concrete walls—impregnated, over the years, with phenol-based disinfectants and urine—served as much more than functional barriers to the wind and rain. Their pungent smell characterized years of deprivation, oppressiveness, disempowerment, and hopelessness, and the rank atmosphere represented only too clearly the frustrations of those who lived and worked inside the walls.

We were all victims; the worst victims, needless to say, were those who had been imprisoned because of their disabilities. They could not escape. They could not go home each day to the beauty of a fragrant herb garden, or to the refreshing air of the salt sea. They could not experience the uplifting of the spirit as a loved one greeted them at the door. Instead, they remained (and some still do, despite our policies of deinstitutionalization) locked inside a world of ugliness; an ugliness that is far removed from the ideal caring environments of Florence Nightingale (1859), Martha Rogers (1970), or Jean Watson (1979); an ugliness that penetrates their very *being* and ultimately destroys their spirit. This ugliness, I regret to say, is perpetuated by poor nursing practice, uncaring management strategies, and a world languishing in its capacity to *care for itself.*

Inside the hospital where I worked, there were over eight hundred individuals, all of whom had varying degrees of intellectual and physical impairment. Each person shared meals, dormitories, and sparse recreation rooms with thirty to fifty fellow residents. The days, for those inside, were filled with myriad experiences of intense emotion: grief, love (rare though it was), anger (much more common), violence, a numbing acceptance, and, for some, profound periods of great learning.

Upon entering this world, one could sense the defeat of a nurse as she knelt to clean the cold, damp surface of the bathroom floor or surveyed the rank and soiled clothes hanging from a despairing man standing nearby. It was the third time that morning that she had washed and changed him, and it was the third time that morning she had yelled at him and ridiculed him because of his disabilities. The frustration and anger, the tears, and the numbing acceptance of the young man echoed hauntingly against the brick walls. Where had the "caring" gone?

Why did a doctor order a nurse and four other workers to hold down a blind girl while the doctor, roughly and untidily, used thick black thread to suture a cut above the girl's eyebrow? There was no anesthetic, despite the girl's struggles and cries of pain. It was the second time that day she had fallen and cut her head on the hard concrete floor, and, for the second time that day, she had been delivered into the hands of that doctor. When the nurse complained of the cruelty and begged for some relief, the doctor replied: "Give her some diazepam after it's finished." The reply caused the nurse to weep along with the young girl.

Today, I still remember these and many more painful moments during which the sanctity of human life dissolved into an atmosphere of fear, dread, and revulsion. There were some good moments, however—some rejuvenating moments that refreshed and energized the spirit. For example, I will never forget Craig, a young man with severe physical disabilities, who used to lie on his stomach most of the time. One day, I had some jelly beans and I placed one on Craig's pillow. He struggled for ever so long to retrieve the jelly bean from the pillow so that he could eat it. Just as he finally got the jelly bean to his mouth, it slipped mischievously out of his hand. There was, first, a look of astonishment, then a glimmer of despair, and, finally, a burst of laughter and a friendly wink from Craig as our eyes met and I exclaimed: "Oh NO! you haven't dropped it after all that?" Precious, seemingly small moments they were; but they reconnected me with the spirit of life. They made the overwhelming restrictions of institutional life and the handicap of a twisted body dissolve into the warmth of spiritual harmony.

I still meet with people who have disabilities—usually, but not always outside of traditional institutions. My friends teach me that institutions are not just bricks and mortar. They represent our fears, our locked-away spirits, our diminished dignity, our devaluing of self. They also have shown me how simply the spirit can be cleansed and rejuvenated through an expression of love, caring, warmth, and nurturing.

The Bright Alps project aims to bring people together to share and learn about each other's humanness while surrounded by the natural beauty of the snow country in the alps of Victoria, Australia. The winter snows melt into the fast-flowing Oven's River. The physically beautiful and inspiring alps provide an energizing environment for refreshing and empowering experiences. Each year, a group of young people—students of nursing, students of medicine, and young adults with intellectual and physical disabilities—visit the alps to spend time with each other and to nurture each other with the spirit of caring. Each year, it is an empowering and healing experience for us all.

The time together is filled with nervous anticipation, laughter, and friendship. We share the excitement as a young woman sees snow for the first time and exclaims at its beauty as it falls softly and silently into the silvery snow gum trees. We laugh at our own clumsiness as we tumble downhill after falling from a crazy toboggan.

Around the fire at night, we find time for reflection and personal reevaluation. Even the young autistic boy who has been pulling our hair continually over the past three days sits quietly and is still in the meditative silence. It is a time for talking of new hopes and dreams, a time for new understandings, a time spent far away from *institutional life* (and I mean that in its broadest sense). It is a most precious time to us all.

This is a simple project, a mere gesture to reaffirm our humanness. Through its experience, we teach each other about ourselves.

PERSONAL STATEMENT

Susan Elsom was born in Australia in 1951 and grew up in a happy, stable, and religious family environment. She was admitted on scholarship to Sydney University, where she undertook a Bachelor of Arts degree. Although she did not complete this degree, she spent one year of further study at a teacher training college and became a teacher of English literature in a country secondary school.

During her university years, she was actively involved in protest marches against the mining of uranium and the production of what was known as "yellow cake," a substance used in the manufacture of nuclear weapons. She also attended peace marches calling for a moratorium on the atrocities committed against people in Vietnam.

In the mid-1970s, she undertook a 600-km bicycle ride through New South Wales with a group of environmentalists called Friends of the Earth (now incorporated with Greenpeace). The finale of the bicycle ride was a "down to earth festival" at Canberra, where people sang and danced together, bathed in the open without clothes, and shared knowledge and skills about natural therapies and living skills.

Her religious background taught her to value human life, and she remains an impassioned advocate for the rights of people who are being mistreated or abused. In 1979, she began a nursing career, caring for people with mental retardation. The experience of institutional life was one of the most shocking, yet empowering experiences of her life.

She is presently a teacher at The Caroline Chisholm School of Nursing, Monash University, and her experiences of the past influence greatly her understanding of the nature and purpose of nursing. She hopes to continue to write and learn about nursing and to undertake research studies in the near future.

REFERENCES

Nightingale, Florence. (1980). *Notes on nursing: What it is and what it is not.* Edinburgh: Churchill Livingstone. (Original published 1859.)

Rogers, M. E. (1970). *An introduction to the theoretical basis of nursing.* Philadelphia: Davis.

Watson, J. (1985). *Nursing: Human science and human care.* Norwalk, CT: Appleton-Century-Crofts.

Wolfensberger, W. (1985). Social role valorization: A new insight, and a new term, for normalization. *AAMR Journal, 9*(1), 5–11.

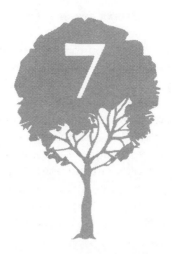

Toward a More Friendly Social Environment for the Patient: The Role of the Resident Hospital Relative

Selina Rwashana

Entry into any hospital around the world is like a transition onto another planet. Not only is the patient met by cold white-clad people who seem ready to administer painful injections at the slightest excuse, but he or she is cut off from the familiar environment outside the hospital.

The evolution of a friendlier social environment in my country, Uganda, has been thrown at us largely out of necessity. A walk down the corridor of any ward in a hospital in Uganda, deep in the night, will reveal that the ward is home both for the patient on the hospital bed and for a close relative, usually found on a mattress beside the patient.

This is evidence of a situation that has evolved out of Uganda's lack of adequate nursing services. Uganda, a country of 17 million people, had, by May 1992, a total of 5,631 nurses (see Table 7–1). A Ugandan midwife attends to 15,000 expectant mothers, and a nurse attends to between 8,000 and 10,000 patients.

Given the above statistics, there is no way a nursing service could operate. As a result, a cadre of nursing service providers has to be developed to complement the work of the nurses.

The person who has become a fixture at patients' bedsides in our hospitals is called the resident hospital relative (RHR)—usually, a spouse, parent, aunt, uncle, brother, grandmother, or other relative close to the patient.

In this chapter, I will highlight the role of the RHR, which has heretofore been ignored. I think the role of a resident hospital relative has to be studied and appreciated in order to render a more socially friendly environment to our patients.

A brief look at this cadre of nursing service providers shows that it evolved as a direct result of inadequacies in the traditional health service. Following independence and the subsequent political turmoil that our country went through, the nurses, like any other professionals, got their share of the problems. Many of the nurses who had undergone training in Britain left Uganda. The few who remained, and those being turned out by our nursing schools, opted for the higher-paying private practice in the drug shops and midwifery homes.

Table 7–1   Uganda's Nursing Profession, May 1992

Chief Nursing Officer	1
Deputy Chief Nursing Officer	1
Principal Nursing Officer	2
Senior Nursing Officer, Grade I	7
Senior Nursing Officer, Grade II	54
Nursing Officer, Grade I	96
Nursing Officer, Grade II	1,571
Enrolled Nurses	2,447
Enrolled Midwives	1,419
Acting Principal Tutors	2
Nurse/Midwifery Tutor	31
Total	5,631

The few nurses who were left to staff the hospitals lost morale because of the ever-increasing cost of living. In our hospitals, nursing staff was not only inadequate but also poorly motivated. The resident hospital relative (RHR) became welcome in meeting this inadequacy.

RHRs have now become part of the hospital establishment. In most hospitals, they are issued special permits that allow them to be in the hospital. Some hospitals, such as Rubaga Hospital, a missionary hospital in Kampala, have gone as far as constructing a structure for RHRs' use. The building is called *Ekijanjabi* (house for helper) in one of the local dialects.

RHRs help in the bathing of the patient, toilet procedures, timely taking of treatment, and preparation of food for the patient. They also act as a link between the hospital staff and the other relatives of the patient. This is important when certain drugs and investigation cannot be provided in the hospital but are available from private practitioners and laboratories.

Socially, the RHRs provide security to the patient who, upon admission to the hospital, experiences a new and cold environment. The people who remain with the patient during the period of the treatment in the hospital will maintain the contact after discharge. This provides a cadre of people who have the patient's confidence and trust and are therefore in a position to influence behavioral change if indicated. This is particularly desirable with treatment of certain conditions where behavioral change is important—alcoholism, hypertension, and diabetes mellitus. For children, the RHRs provide a group of people who are readily educatable in the prevention of malnutrition and diarrheal diseases and their related complications. This is because the RHR is usually the mother, who witnesses how high-energy and protein foods (for malnutrition) and oral rehydration salt solutions (in dehydration) have healed their children.

In our struggle to provide a more socially friendly environment, we should appreciate, educate, and render appropriate skills to this cadreship. They are essential to remedy the inadequacies in our current nursing service.

PART

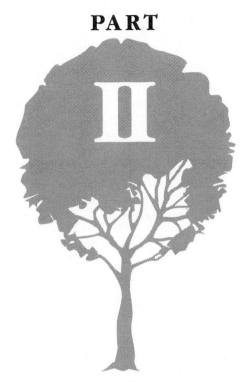

II

Environment in Practice Perspectives

This Part highlights the dynamic interplay of (a) the interior life of the self in creating environmentally responsible nursing practice with (b) the exterior environments. A clear message shines through in these chapters. We are our environments. In this part, authors describe ways of bringing environmental consciousness into the world of everyday nursing practice. We invite you to peruse the ways nurses live their commitment to environmentally responsible practice as you read through this part.

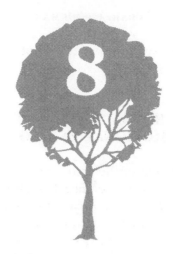

The Emotional Environment of Older Adults: A Holistic Nursing Perspective*

Craig A. Cookman

I would like to share with you a few of my ideas about environmental connections relevant to the health and well-being of older adults. In so doing, I offer a beginning description of environment from a perspective focused on the emotional, heartfelt connections the older person experiences in everyday life, rather than on his or her physical surroundings. After outlining how the emotional environment is described, I shall develop six dimensions of this environment and show how they may function to

*I would like to acknowledge the support from the National Center for Nursing Research, National Institutes of Health, Award #NR06482, for the research that made the ideas presented here possible.

form a holistic representation of the emotional environment of older people.

DESCRIPTION AND FUNCTION OF
THE EMOTIONAL ENVIRONMENT

To consider the concept of the emotional environment, we must resist the natural tendency to comprehend the environment from an objective or "other" perspective and instead allow ourselves to share the person's subjective experience. To elicit information on this subjective experience, I have interviewed older adults about aspects of the environment they "feel close to" or "feel connected to." I have also found it useful to ask people what they are "attached to," as a way of eliciting information on this subjective environment.

The emotional environment can be defined as a domain of everyday experience involving interactions with people, places, things, animals, and ideas a person feels "close to" or "connected to"—all of which may be described as attachments. The emotional environment functions as a supportive structure that promotes a sense of identity, belonging, and connectedness, a buffer against the effects of loneliness and feelings of depression. The emotional environment gives us "someone," or "something," or "somewhere" to turn for help when needed. In a sense, the emotional environment gives us a sense of purpose by forming the structure that contains the people and things we care about.

DIMENSIONS OF THE EMOTIONAL ENVIRONMENT

The dimensions of the emotional environment are formed by the categories of objects (as used in the generic sense—meaning persons, places, things, or ideas) a person feels "close to" or expresses an "attachment to." In an everyday sense, when we say we feel an attachment to our family members, friends, and other objects such as our home, we are speaking of objects in the domain of the emotional environment. I categorize that environment into six dimensions: (1) people, (2) groups of people, (3) things, (4) animals, (5) places, and (6) ideas.

People

The most easily recognized dimension of the emotional environment of older people (and other developmental phases of the life span as well) are "significant others," including family and friends. People—children, parents, and grandparents (to name a few)— function to give the older person roles and the associated identity afforded by those roles. Being a grandparent can give the older person a "sense of being needed" as a source of wisdom, advice, and nurturance in times of stress. The people in the emotional environment serve to define supportive, meaningful, and worthwhile functions where assistance is both given and received. The roles and supportive functions provided by people as a dimension of the emotional environment can be valuable connections in everyday life because they diminish feelings of aloneness and promote a sense of well-being.

Groups of People

In addition to individual others, belonging to groups of people defines a dimension of the emotional environment. Being a member of a church group or a community organization provides a connectedness that can contribute to a sense of identity for the older person. Groups of people is included as a dimension of the emotional environment because it is usually the concept of "the group" to which older adults express an attachment. Individual group members may come and go, but the group is often the important distinction that defines the emotional tie and gives the older person a sense of purpose and belonging.

Things

A third dimension of the emotional environment for older people is things—objects of an inanimate nature toward which older people express feelings of closeness and attachment. For many older people whom I have interviewed, things remain a significant dimension of their emotional attachments, although a less important dimension than at earlier (i.e., younger) times. For many, retirement involved a move from a larger home where they raised their families to an apartment or a mobile home. Because this change usually involved a move to smaller quarters, many possessions were handed down to children or sold. Certain possessions were kept because of the memories associated with them—family photos, trophies indicative of past accomplishments, or heirlooms. Other researchers (Wallendorf & Arnould, 1988; Sherman & Newman, 1977–1978) have found declines in the liking of favorite things past age 65. Many of the older people I interviewed attributed a lack of attachment to material things to their being raised during the poverty-stricken Great Depression years.

Animals

Animals, especially companion animals (pets), are a great source of emotional comfort and support for some older people. In an earlier study (Cookman, 1988), I interviewed five older adults about the attachment they felt toward their newly adopted pet dogs. These older people described coming to a time when they became aware that their lives felt empty and hollow; they had intense feelings of loneliness and a general lack of purpose and connectedness in life. Pet adoption provided "someone" to communicate with, "someone" to come to know and understand, and "someone" to be with and share everyday life with. I used the phrase "filling the void" to describe how these pet dogs functioned within the emotional environment of these older people. Pet animals are widely used in visitation programs to institutional populations of older people, to stimulate the senses and promote socialization in these settings. At least for some older adults, animals contribute a valuable dimension to the emotional environment.

Places

A fifth dimension of the emotional environment of older people refers to the geographical places held as "close"—places that elicit feelings of attachment and closeness. A great deal of research has tried to identify which groups of older people will exhibit "migratory" retirement patterns, and which groups will "age in place," citing that they have "put down roots" in a particular home, neighborhood, or town, and wish to stay. The issue here is not which persons are "migrators" and which are "rooted"; rather, it is to recognize that places are an important dimension of the emotional environment that has relevance for the behavior and well-being of older people. We have learned much over the past 20 years about the trauma involved in relocation from one place to another—usually from independent living at home to some form of institutional setting. What is missing from current knowledge is information about the loss of a dimension of this emotional environment. Can this dimension be substituted for? Grieved for and then substituted for? Ever established again? Transformed to a new attachment to the former place? Questions such as these can be addressed by examination of the environment from an emotional perspective such as the one described here, but answers are difficult to reach using an outsider's viewpoint.

Ideas

Ideas represent the last of the six dimensions of the emotional environment I will describe here. I am using the term to include thoughts, beliefs, values, memories, imagination, and fantasy, and perhaps other experiences that occur within the consciousness of the older person. The notion that a person's ideas, beliefs, or memories may represent "objects" that evoke feelings of closeness and connectedness in later life is one that requires careful consideration and study. If it is true, as suggested in the literature on adult development, that people become increasingly introspective in later life (Schaie & Willis, 1986), then coping strategies referred to as "passive mastery"—contemplation, reflection, and self-evaluation, for example—deserve consideration as relevant environmental concepts for older adults. There is essentially no research to consult that examines the subjective, contemplative, inner worlds of older people from an emotional perspective. Observing older people gazing out a window for long periods of time, I have often wondered:

"What are they thinking about? Is this the behavior of a bored person—or is some important cognitive process occurring?" In my earlier study (Cookman, 1992), 68% of a sample of community-living older adults indicated they could feel "close" to memories or other ideas. Perhaps if we were to become more willing to accept a child's "imaginary friend" as a developmental ally, we might also embrace excursions of the imagination in the healthy development of older persons.

INDIVIDUAL DIFFERENCES AND AGE-RELATED CHANGES FROM AN EMOTIONAL ENVIRONMENT PERSPECTIVE

Defining these six dimensions of the emotional environment can appear to restrict the variability and individuality of a person's subjective interpretation of his or her emotional environment without further explanation. In this section, I will outline how individual and group (in this case, age-group) differences can be accounted for, using the emotional environment perspective.

Individual Differences

Individuals can indicate great variability in the way they exhibit the six dimensions of the emotional environment. The simplest example I can think of is the case of those who choose not to own pets, or may even relate a distaste for animals altogether. It would be tempting to say that this dimension was not relevant for them. Might we even say that this dimension of the emotional environment is not relevant for everyone? Do those who choose to form emotional attachments to pet animals simply have the usual dimensions "plus this other one"?

My answer would be that they have a distinctive interaction with animals as a dimension of their emotional environment—an interaction that hasn't involved, and perhaps shouldn't involve, contact with animals. People who have had lifelong allergies to pet hair are one example. I would, however, continue to assert that the relevance of this dimension of their emotional environment is equivalent to that of the person who expresses great feelings of closeness to a pet. The dimension has a different expression; its absence or presence is not at issue. Individuals can therefore differ with respect to the amount of emotional energy they invest in each of the six dimensions. Some dimensions will contribute more to their sense of identity and connectedness than will others. There is no end to the unique expressions of the six dimensions of this view of the emotional environment.

Age-Related Changes

Older people, as a group, have some characteristics that seem to be related to retirement and other later-life issues. I would like to point out a couple of these so that the emotional environment perspective doesn't appear to be so concrete as to have relevance only to description of individuals. As I noted earlier, in my description of things as a dimension of the emotional environment, attachment to things as inanimate objects appears to decline with age. One study found that it declines sharply past age 65 (Wallendorf & Arnould, 1988). It may be that older people as a group derive few supportive benefits in this dimension. It may be helpful to assist older people in the appropriate "handing down" of things while preserving the subset of objects that the older person desires to keep. Similarly, it would appear that memories or other ideas seem to gain importance with age. Programs that teach reminiscence or life-review skills and strategies may enhance this dimension, thereby leading to an increased sense of well-being and connectedness. The provision of time to be alone to think may be as important as socialization programs in meeting attachment needs and environmental connections.

A Model of Connections to the Emotional Environment

I have prepared three models of the emotional environment. Each model depicts a different environmental expression; two represent different individuals, and one is a possible model of later life. I will highlight what each model indicates in terms of differences in emphasis among the dimensions, and will point to ways in which these depictions could be used to approach an increased understanding of the individual or group.

The model depicted in Figure 8-1 shows the six dimensions of the emotional environment as a pie chart, with each of the slices representing one of the dimensions. In this representation, all slices are the same size, indicating that this individual has an equal emphasis, in terms of emotional involvement, with all six dimensions. This person is very diverse, in that all dimensions are represented equally, but because the people connections for this person do not exceed the emphasis placed on animals, places, or things, this may not be an extremely social person. An increased understanding of this person's emotional environment emerges from the model and may indicate relating differently to this person, depending on the situation.

The model in Figure 8-2 depicts a very different individual. The slice of the pie representing attachments to individuals is much larger than any of the other dimensions. The portion for groups of

Figure 8–1   Emotional Environment Model:
Individual Profile 1

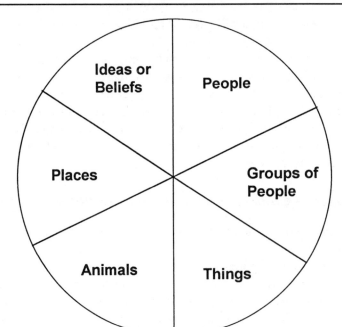

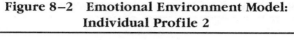

**Figure 8–2   Emotional Environment Model:
Individual Profile 2**

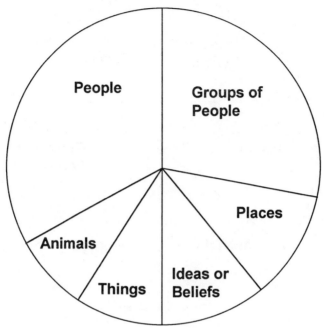

people is also very large, and the other dimensions occupy a relatively small area of the model. This person is a "people person"
who prefers a lot of socialization and interaction in groups. Interaction with animals is of minimal interest, as is having much time
alone. This person has a different emotional environment profile,
compared to the person represented in Figure 8-1.

The model in Figure 8-3 is intended to reflect older adults as a
group. The sizes of the slices are arbitrarily assigned and do not
represent specific proportions; they are shown here to highlight
differences in emphasis that may apply among older adults. The
people and ideas or beliefs dimensions are much larger than the
others, although each of the others remains significant. A very important distinction regarding older adults is made here: Certain
dimensions of the environment declined, but others expanded to
preserve the environment as a healthy, nondisengaging, growth-
enabling view of development and aging. The environment itself

Figure 8–3   Emotional Environment Model: Group Profile 1

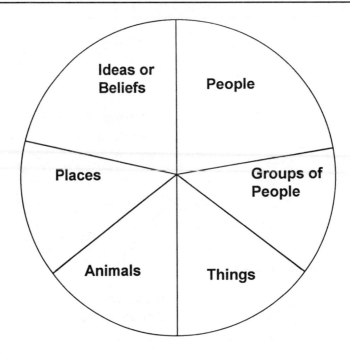

is not diminished; rather, it is undergoing developmental change and transformation.

This generalized depiction of both individuals and groups serves as an example of how the emotional environment may be defined and used. More interesting series of models could be constructed to depict changes with age within an individual—perhaps in five-year increments across the life span, or between groups of individuals in different health states.

SUMMARY AND CONCLUSION

This chapter has presented a broad description of what I have termed the emotional environment of older people. Six dimensions of the emotional environment have been defined: (1) people, (2) groups of people, (3) things, (4) animals, (5) places, and

(6) ideas. How to address both individual and group differences, within this framework, was discussed and illustrated. Two individual emotional environment profiles and one profile depicting older adults as a group were presented as examples of how individual and group profiles could describe different individuals and groups based on the emotional environment model.

Current knowledge about the role and function of the environment in regard to the health of older people is largely concerned with issues of safety. Most gerontological nursing textbooks describe environmental concerns in terms of protecting the older person from his or her surroundings; the environment should be clean, uncluttered, and free from risk of injury and disease. Although these concerns are extremely important and represent essential areas of attention, we need to move into more holistic views that recognize the supportive functions of the environment.

The environment is intrinsically neither a villain nor an ally; it simply *is.* Aging does create increased safety concerns, but the opportunities for growth through interactions with the environment seem also to be enhanced. We need to explore our connections with the environment to define a more balanced view wherein the challenges presented by the environment are balanced with its supportive opportunities.

PERSONAL STATEMENT

My interest in environmental concerns began when I worked with my grandparents, who owned and operated Oxbow Rest Home in rural Newbury, Vermont. At age five or six, I carried meal trays to the six or seven older adult residents of the home, and did other "errands" appropriate for a young nurse in training. I have very fond memories of spending time with the residents. "Peppy" (probably age 85 or so) used to take me fishing with him, and we worked in the garden—sometimes pulling weeds but always looking for fishworms. A delightful woman (older than Peppy!) who used to live in "the front room" taught me how to score Red Sox baseball games. She watched every game and, I'm sure, kept better statistics than the official scorer. The residents ate vegetables from the garden—fresh in season, and canned during most of the winter.

Since that early orientation, I have always enjoyed working with older people and have pursued gerontological nursing as a career. My particular interests have included the role of pet animals in promoting the mental health of older people, and the maintenance of our natural connections with the environment as a pattern of healthy human functioning. It is my hope that knowledge about the role of the environment in matters of health will become a priority in the 1990s and beyond, as I believe it once was.

REFERENCES

Cookman, C. A. (1988). *Filling the void: A descriptive study of the process of attachment between elderly people and their pets.* Unpublished master's thesis, University of Arizona.

Cookman, C. A. (1992). Attachment structures of older adults: Theory development using a mixed qualitative–quantitative research design. Doctoral dissertation, University of Arizona. *Dissertation Abstracts International, 53*(7B), 3398.

Schaie, K. W., & Willis, S. L. (1986). *Adult development and aging. British Journal of Psychiatry, 133,* 550–555.

Sherman, E., & Newman, E. (1977–1978). The meaning of cherished personal possessions for the elderly. *Journal of Aging and Human Development, 8*(2), 181–192.

Wallendorf, M., & Arnould, E. J. (1988). "My favorite things": A cross-cultural inquiry into object attachment, possessiveness, and social linkage. *Journal of Consumer Research, 14,* 531–547.

Encountering Environment
through Interiority

Marilyn A. Ray

Reflection on papers on ecological nursing presented at the first international conference on nursing and the environment illuminates the depth of awareness of human-environment interconnection, and our new dialogue with nature (Capra & Steindl-Rast, with Matus, 1991). This celebration of belongingness—to the environment, to each other, and to the spirit of the universe—has recaptured the best of our intellectual history, from premodern thought, through modernism, to the new postmodern relational thinking of today. These three historical periods have contributed to the view of dynamic responsibility now occurring in the world: (1) the premodern view of holism, which located human beings at the center of the cosmos and the spiritual realm; (2) the modern period of empirical science, which contributed causality and critical rationality; and (3) the present images of the postmodern world, which are historical, participatory, and personal (Miller, 1989). The door to a deeper and richer understanding and to an accountability for the recognition of human-environment interdependency has been opened.

The personal-mutual sense of community emerging in the universe (Kirkpatrick, 1986) presents a challenge to both the Copernican cosmology, which placed the solar system in a dominant role at the center of the universe, and the Cartesian perspective of the self as separate and distinct from the world (Tarnas, 1991). Merleau-Ponty (1962) reminded us that our environment is the only place where we truly know ourselves. We seek meaning by looking at the world as we meet it in immediate experience. We speak about our relationship to the world in language shaped by reflective inquiry into what it means to function—to know, value, deliberate, and decide—in the world (Lonergan cited in Webb, 1988). In essence, the human-environment relationship is the scope of experience as seen upon reflection. Polanyi (1958/1961) called this intellectual function personal knowing, and Lonergan (1970; Webb, 1988) called it self-reflective consciousness or interiority. In the postmodern world, ". . . all knowing is [considered] personal; that is, dependent upon a commitment of the knower within a community of value" (Miller, 1989, p. 12). In this chapter, I focus on recovering this commitment of the knower to a community of value by interpreting the meaning of encountering the environment through interiority—interiority of the soul through personal reflections on actions within the world.

COMMITMENT TO A COMMUNITY OF VALUE

Despite awareness of human-environment interconnection and the quest for a new communitarianism, the atomistic views of the modern period in science, technology, economics, and politics continue to maintain a hold on our thought. Subsequently, atomistic thought continues to influence our values and social institutions, where the impetus for an ecological consciousness gets its start. We witness the evils of the destabilization of values and cultures, and the promotion of unrealistic expectations of commercialism and consumerism (Henderson, 1988). Frequently, we look to what we perceive as powerful to save a society. For example, we often perceive economics as powerful. However, traditional economics, by fostering competition and greed instead of cooperation and relational ethics, fails to enable institutions to choose an ecological philosophy (Henderson, 1988).

In a recent book, *The Good Society,* Bellah, Madsen, Sullivan, Swidler, and Tipton (1991) remarked on the efforts needed to create good institutions, good communities, and a good society. The authors explained that all actions are responses to action upon us, that is, responsibility. By responsibility they mean our inescapable connection to a web of relationship with others, the natural world, and God. Along with acting responsibly comes the idea of personal accountability. Accountability is an ethic of concern characterizing accountability whereby we pay attention to our effect on others and the environment. This means considering what we do and how we act, as well as the consequences of our actions. The authors (Bellah et al., 1991) concluded that the key to acting responsibly and with accountability is trust and reliance on trustworthiness. In effect, when enough of us have sufficient trust to act responsibly, there is a chance to achieve, at least in part, the creation of moral institutions and, ultimately, a good society.

A LOOK INWARD TO THE SOUL

Reflection on the goals of this environmental conference and the theme of *The Good Society* (Bellah et al., 1991) calls for attention not only to what we do, but also to who we are. Is it possible to truthfully herald the tenets of ecological nursing—protection and care for the environment—without first looking inward to the state of one's soul? Like Moore (1992), in my view, a dynamic ecology, while requiring empathetic participation with others to create new economies, technologies, and essentially a new trustworthiness within communities and institutions, requires first "centering within oneself and looking into the soul as the means to cultivate sacredness in everyday life" (Moore, 1992). "The soul suffers more from the everyday conditions of life when they do not nourish it with the solid experiences it craves" (Moore, 1992, p. 209). Moore (1992) claims the soul craves care. Care of the soul ". . . is an appreciation of the paradoxical mysteries that blend light and darkness into the grandeur of what human life and culture can be" (Moore, 1992, p. xix). Self-reflection is the means to appreciation.

Psalm 51 (1993) states:

> . . . *Create in me a clean heart, O God; and renew a right spirit within me . . . . (p. 43)*

The psalmist, David, prays to God to create in him a clean heart. He declares that truth and righteousness are in the inward soul where wisdom dwells.

Praying for the creation of a clean heart illuminates the need for an authentic relationship between the interior life and outward action. For a life to be lived in relation to what one truly loves or desires to change (care of the environment or the human–environment relationship) requires also a language of love and ethical transformation within the self. Genuine longings cannot be discovered in a purely objective sense by looking only outward to the world but by subjective existence constituted by intentional operations of self-critical reflection and self-transcending love (Webb, 1988). "[V]irtue [however] is never genuine when it sets itself apart from evil" (Moore, 1992, p. 134). Virtue is only understood in concert with evil. This "existential tension" or "synthesis between the infinite and finite" (philosophical perspectives put forth by Voegelin and Kierkegaard, respectively (Webb, 1988, p. 286)), illuminate the constant struggle of the human heart—the dialectic between the impulse to destroy (doing evil), and the impulse to transform (doing good). Attunement to the soul and prayers for renewal of a right spirit permit revelation of deep meaning toward the right action to be released in daily life.

We often witness the paradox of ecological evil and good in the current culture. Attempting to harness good aims (environmental care) by appealing to lower motives (negative or hostile models of power) will not effectively reduce the evil of neglect. Promoting good will only happen when people do not return evil for evil.

"Evil cannot soil genuine goodness and purity; it cannot defile it. It causes good people to suffer, but because of their suffering and their refusal to pass it on, evil vanishes" (Allen, 1989, p. 34).

CONCLUSION

The unfailing truth that springs forth from care of the soul is love and relatedness which, in turn, allows for a certain way of living—caring about everything because, we, in essence, belong together. "Relatedness is a signal of soul" (Moore, 1992, p. 94), a signal of love, and it dignifies all love, including love of the environment.

Let us hope that, within the global agenda of environmental caring, there will be the impetus for continued leadership toward trustworthiness—a deep spiritual and ecological flowing together. Interconnectedness or belongingness is a response to the interior life of the soul and to the creation of human communities. Capra (Capra & Steindl-Rast, with Matus, 1991) remarked that "[i]f an ecological life is ultimately a spiritual life, then it becomes a spiritual discipline" (p. 177). Thus, to the extent that we are first liberated in our souls, that is, fully alive, we are then disciplined to be responsive to the challenges needed for effective and sustained environmental action.

PERSONAL STATEMENT

My interest in environment was motivated by the first Earth Day celebration in San Francisco in the early 1970s. Californians were particularly concerned about the damage to the environment by auto pollutants, and the need to preserve the beauty of the Pacific shoreline and the exquisite fauna, flora, and wildlife of the area. From this initial motivation, I have taught a form of ecological nursing to undergraduate and graduate students in all my courses.

My philosophical and research interests center around caring. Recently, I developed a philosophical view of complex caring dynamics illuminating human–environment interconnectedness and choice making as the focus of nursing inquiry. To more fully understand the responsibilities of human–environment integrality, I place special emphasis on interiority, a deep, personal, and intuitive knowing that calls forth listening to the voice of God within. This, in turn, facilitates communicating the language of love in word and deed. My commitment is to persist relentlessly in encouraging reflection on the ethics of interiority and authenticity as a means to facilitate collective action toward protection and care of all living creatures and the environment.

REFERENCES

Allen, D. (1989). Christian values in a post-Christian context. *Postmodern theology*. San Francisco: Harper/San Francisco.

Bellah, R., Madsen, R., Sullivan, W., Swidler, A., Tipton, S. (1991). *The good society*. New York: Alfred A. Knopf.

Capra, F., & Steindl-Rast, D., with Matus, T. (1991). *Belonging to the universe*. San Francisco: Harper/San Francisco.

Henderson, H. (1988). *Politics of the solar age: Alternatives to economics*. Indianapolis: Knowledge Systems.

Kirkpatrick, F. (1986). *Community: A trinity of models*. Washington, DC: Georgetown University Press.

Lonergan, B. (1970). *Insight: A study of human understanding* (3rd ed.). New York: Philosophical Library.

Merleau-Ponty, M. (1962). *Phenomenology of perception*. London: Routledge & Kegan Paul.

Miller, J. (1989). *The emerging postmodern world: Postmodern theology*. San Francisco: Harper/San Francisco.

Moore, T. (1992). *Care of the soul*. New York: HarperCollins.

Polanyi, M. (1958/1961). *Personal knowledge*. Chicago: The University of Chicago Press.

Psalm 51. (1993). *The book of Psalms*. New York: Dover.

Tarnas, R. (1991). *The passion of the Western mind*. New York: Ballantine Books.

Webb, E. (1988). *Philosophers of consciousness*. Seattle: The University of Washington Press.

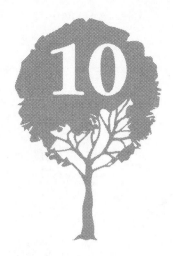

A Collage of Awareness for a Sustainable Future

Carolyn L. Brown

Commitment to environmental concerns and to preserving a future that will sustain life starts with awareness. From awareness flow the many ways of creating healthy environments. Just thinking about the word *environment* brings forth a multitude of images that assault my senses. Daily, screaming headlines greet me (see p. 120).

What frightens me is that I truly believe that I am my environment, in that I am formed of earth elements, taking in and giving out healthy and noxious particles constantly. I am what surrounds me. Because so much of what I am aware of in my environment is noxious, and I know it is part of me, what saves me is that knowing often operates outside my awareness. In most of my everyday life, I live in a state of unawareness. But when the awareness surfaces again, so does the dis-ease and fear as I search for ways to find health, peace, and harmony.

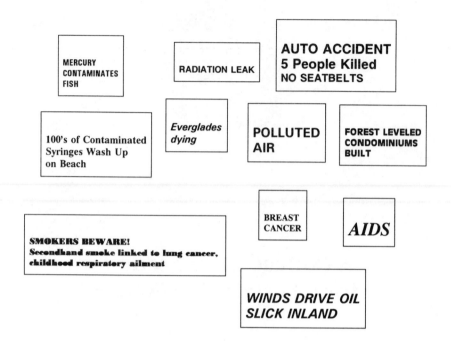

I know the environment from many perspectives. Because my abilities to perceive are finite, I know only parts of the fabric of the environment at any given point in time. I view the environment from many different standpoints: parent, citizen, woman, nurse, administrator, person, consumer, friend; all are entangled, but they still originate from the whole person that is me. As I become more aware, more attuned, my senses open to what surrounds me. Poetry, as a sort of photography of the mind-world mixed with the environment-world, serves me best as a way to express my awareness of environment. Three poems evolved as awareness unfolded in a deeper, more personal way. Each poem tells its own story from the perspective of a different role—friend, nurse, and outraged person.

FIRST POEM

The first poem involves the sad story of a good friend, now dead. My husband, Tom, and I have known Don and his family for over

19 years. Tom and Don were both Army Social Workers; Don was Tom's "boss." Gradually, he and his family became our friends. Don, father of four teenagers then, was full of energy and deeply religious; he lived values of caring for others. A huge man, he was gentle and kind. Over the years, we maintained contact. While not closest friends, something always drew us together, creating a bond that withstood separation and time. In 1992, I went to the Northwest for a conference, and visited Don and his family. His fifth child, born soon after our son was born, was now 16, and Don was dying. Don used to stand about six-foot-five, with a massive frame to match his height. Now, shrunken with illness, he was eyeball to eyeball with me, and I stand about five-foot-two. Still the sweet smile, but the pain and anger at what was happening to him were clear. He was determined to live one more year, to see his son graduate from high school. We made plans that year to get together as couples and go on a cruise. To our amazement, we learned they were coming to visit in February 1993, traveling by cruise ship. When they docked in Ft. Lauderdale, Don's appearance shocked us. He was even smaller and frailer, as if he were shrinking his body until it became too small to house him anymore. We talked, laughed, and shared stories, with the sadness and tears tucked away behind our eyelids. They were to stay four days, but their visit was cut short by Don's inability to breathe. He needed to get back to see his doctor. What does his story have to do with environmental issues? In the following poem, I believe the connection is clear. Most likely, Don died early and painfully because we humans do not create environments that sustain life.

Don

My friend of many years
I see you in a long-ago day
Tall, straight, sweet welcoming smile
moving quickly and surely through your days of
family
friends
church
duty to country . . .
helping others.

Now I see you
hunched over in chair too large for your shrinking frame,
vertebrae and bones crumbling
head sunken unto chest with body a painful curve,
    can't sit up and can't lie down,
gasping for breath
drowning in fluid from lungs
    unable to bear the pain of
    coughing. . . .

Now you look up as I pass
I see your sweet fragile smile
and ask,
"How are you doing?"
at three a.m.
Can't sleep, you or me.
I choke on my own tears.

Why?
Why this broken body with screaming pain?
Why this life too soon to end?
What cause?
Who knows for sure . . .

Living near test site,
    nuclear weapons, above-ground Atomic bombs
    going off in the desert . . .
Fallout assaulting your poor body . . .
Creating your pain today???
Maybe

The army calls you
    to live among cigarette smoke in the
    hazy blue rings of multiple staff meetings,
    and other meetings . . .
and calls you to go to Viet Nam
    with agent orange
    agent sleeping 'til later death.
Creating your pain today???
Maybe

Again you are called by duty
* to live near smokestack tall,*
* spewing toxic, terrible, nefarious smoke*
* until it smokes no more*
* shut down by outrage.*
Creating your pain today???
Maybe

Persons' indifference to life
* caring for personal gain*
* for winning*
Robbed me of your friendship.

I will miss the love
stolen from me
from us
by materials created for gain
* for destruction.*

The warmth of your joy
ripped away by assault from
by products of
* greed*
* neglect*
* hostility*
* arrogance*
* disdain*
ripped away by assault on
* body, mind, spirit*
* all one*
* all you*
* all going*
* too soon to be gone.*

The poetry ends here. Three months later, we learned Don had died. He did not see his son graduate, nor his wife cared for by a secure pension, nor his grandchildren growing up. Who knows why he had cancer; but I believe his body responded to multiple environmental insults by shutting down defenses. His cells, confused by environmental assault, began to act erratically and no longer fulfilled their orderly functions. I believe we all killed Don through our indifference to environmental concerns.

SECOND POEM

As a nurse and faculty member, I took undergraduate students into clinical settings where I was aware of environment in a different way. One of these places was hotel-beautiful, in perfectly matched colors, with no warmth to sustain life. It housed mostly old people who needed minimal care. One floor was devoted to those who needed more care; most suffered from advancing Alzheimer's disease. I believe they suffered from a double-edged assault: an advancing physical disease ripping away their minds, and a sterile, cold, uncaring environment. Even well-intentioned staff could not erase the effects of the cold, perfect sterility of a hotellike environment. Everything was perfect, saying "Don't touch." This poem evolved from walking through their world.

Third Floor

Lined up in hallways
broken, sunken men and women
old fragile joyless eyes
waiting for lunch.

Lying in beds
in rooms.
Dreary and clanking noise.
Hurry, rush, dash, and run,
*   ignoring your shout of unspoken need.*

Lights perfect in intensity and coldness.
Colors perfectly coordinated,
*   too dreary to sustain life.*
Music like pablum
*   when you hunger for steak.*
Voices in the hall
*   talking about the score,*
*   the birdie on the golf course.*

And you, at center,
   old and broken
   crave peace and beauty
   for healing, not just curing,
   healing body, mind, and spirit.

From harmony at center
   and outward to the fringe,
   which is us
      and all need
      the warmth
      of disorder and loving touch
      of music that calls to our spirits
      of the invitation to be a part of things
         to create
         love
         shout
         laugh
         and **be with** *one another*
      in our need.

Nurses work in many environments. Often, these environments manifest the epitome of efficiency and hygiene, stripping away any evidence of nurturing the human spirit. Equally often, environments providing "health care" are themselves unhealthy. Ventilation systems circulate pathogens and other noxious materials. Noise levels are well beyond safe levels for preservation of hearing, much less allowing for rest. Color schemes are impersonal, creating space where people feel like uncomfortable strangers or unwanted guests. Often, the interpersonal environment promotes energy shutdown. Energy people could use to heal themselves goes into coping with an unfriendly environment. Others, in need of long-term care, are stored in what feels like a warehouse where they will never be free. Last days on earth are often spent in sterile solitude, bereft of the warmth and energy of caring relationships.

In addition to sterile surroundings, health care workplaces foster the sick values of pushing people, more and more, to do the work with fewer and fewer resources. Corners are cut. Care becomes no frills at best, lacking in essential elements at the least.

People feel as if they work on an assembly line, without the time to see the whole. When one spends too much time on one person, the next may go wanting and become like a Monday or Friday car. Institutions become warehouses for throwaway people.

Health care workers concern themselves with the disparity between what they believe to be optimal care and the economic mandate to cut corners on the quality of care given. What level of care should be the bare minimum? Because health care workers are stretched and stressed to the maximum, they become ill—burned out, or physically or mentally ill when the stress is too great and the control too little. A number of researchers and organizational experts (Barnett, Biener, & Baruch, 1987; Brown, 1991; Fassel, 1990; Karasek & Theorell, 1990; Matteson & Ivancevich, 1987; Rosen, 1991; Schaef & Fassel, 1988) have highlighted the effects of working in environments where people have little control over their work lives. Yet, little has been done to create healthier environments for those who provide care in such organizations. The current work ethic in the United States creates pressure to overwork and join the growing ranks of workaholics (Fassel, 1990). Again, becoming aware allows greater latitude to choose knowingly, rather than blindly react by fulfilling organizational expectations at the expense of self and those who need health care.

THIRD POEM

The last poem, created as a reflection on environment, brings together a multitude of impressions from the standpoint of outraged person, irrespective of role.

Reflections on Environment

Life-giving, life-supporting energy
Life itself
Freeing
Constricting
Calling upon us for healing
Calling upon us for our own becoming

The emotions
The body
The mind
The wind
The soothing green of grass, trees,
sparkling with the life-giving dew of moisture
The wet of life
The wind carrying and intermingling us all.

What is this "environment" thing??

War within ourselves
War within our homes
War within our communities
War within our nations and between our nations
blocking our energy
negating our need to be with one another
Rape *of mind*
Rape *of person*
Rape *of animal life*
Rape *of earth*
injuring us all
blocking our energy
to create harmony and joy among us all
plant, animal, rock, mineral
all of life

Glut *of mind*
overwhelming consciousness
Glut *of waterways*
choking fish,
Glut *of air*
suffocating all,
Glut *of senses,*
overwhelming

with more, *more,* *more!*

and with trash, trash, trash!
poisoning and blocking
our energy
to move freely

Our ways
create sickness
*   in need of healing*
schisms separating self from earth and universe
sores visible and invisible
tissues in rebellion
spirit closing off to save itself
becoming more and more constricted to avoid
ASSAULT
RAPE
GLUT

and bursting forth in ANGER!
in RAPE!
and MURDER!
of other spirit beings
and
of ourselves.

Calling for freedom
to live more simply
aware
with the well-being of one another
in mind, and heart, and soul
freeing the spirit
freeing our energy
to love
each leaf
and fuzzy kitten
and old man with gnarled hand
and newborn being with eyes tight shut
and girl child
and man child

and puppy child
respecting roaches
the warm moistness of earth.

Stop raping and murdering the earth
that supplies our needs.
Stop raping and murdering ourselves
and live now
in harmony with all
live now
in joyful unity
creating

tomorroW

Awareness and consciousness are unusual phenomena for us humans. When so much assails our senses, we become numb as a way of keeping on with everyday life. If we attend to everything around us that calls for corrective action, we become immobilized because we cannot diffuse our energy in so many directions.

How does one choose a direction, or start changing old ways of living, when so much needs changing? With great caution about sounding prescriptive, I suggest not taking action too soon. If we allow ourselves to become fully aware, immersing ourselves in the fullness of experience, the direction for action will emerge clearly. Let the headlines sink in. Let the sounds, sights, and smells of our lives enter our consciousness, becoming a part of us, rather than merely the context for a solitary pursuit of life. Let us become fully aware of connections, recognizing that all that is out there is within us, creating us in an unending cycle.

The person who enters the hospital for cardiac problems—what led to disease? Advertising for cholesterol-inducing foods, pressures from home and work to do more and more with no time for respite or body. To care for self may be to lose one's job, but to keep the job may result in loss of self. Driving alone in freeway traffic to get to work, breathing smog-laden air, listening to loud stock market reports—no time or dollars for adequate health care. Individual choices? Yes *and* no. We engage in socially and culturally prescribed behaviors based on values that no longer work if we intend to sustain the life of the ecosystem. Appropriate action may be to gently increase the awareness of the person experiencing cardiac illness. But another important part of the cycle is to commit to nurse a new client—the environment. Our clients in multiple health care settings call for recognition of environmental connections leading to disease. Healing starts with recognition. As we nurse the environment, our own health will improve, because we are as integrally connected with the environment as those who have already become ill. Through awareness, the way for each of us to create a sustainable future will become clear. Lifestyles, health care organizations, and nursing practices change a little at a time, through awareness of interconnections with the whole ecosystem and conscious daily choices.

PERSONAL STATEMENT

My interest in environmental issues grew from studying power for nurse executives in different health care environments. Nurses and women, including myself, are interested in power issues because we perceive we could be more powerful but we do not know how. For me, the questions became "What is power?" and "Power for what?" Both intrigued me. My definition of power continues to evolve. Right now, it is:

> *[P]ower is a life force, an energy, that is available to us all. It comes to be from choosing how we are with one another in dynamic interaction with the whole. Our choices either constrain or free energy . . . for ourselves, groups, organizations, others. How we enact, and allow others to enact their power, creates the meaning of our work lives, and our very selves. . . . Power comes to be from everyday, minute-by-minute choices based on lived values, rather than by grand design. (Brown, 1994, p. 87)*

Because much of my work is phenomenological, I opened my self to learning from multiple sources. The direction I needed to take became more clear: researching, teaching, and writing. Helping nurses explore multiple opportunities in order to increase their power according to newer definitions; freeing them to explore their environments; and finding ways to modify them toward greater health through their educational experience—these goals provide the avenue for my work toward a healthier ecosystem. In other areas of my life, life-style changes come slowly but surely, beginning with increasing awareness. I give myself and my family permission to be imperfect as we change. As we do these things, we even have fun, something I recommend for all of us.

REFERENCES

Barnett, R. C., Biener, L, & Baruch, G. (Eds.). (1987). *Gender and stress.* New York: Free Press.

Brown, C. (1991). Health, energy and power as experienced by nurses in their everyday work lives. *Journal of Holistic Nursing, 9*(3), 48–56.

Brown, C. (1994). Power for midlife women: Written on the breeze. In P. Munhall (Ed.), *In women's experience.* New York: National League for Nursing.

Fassel, D. (1990). *Working ourselves to death: The high cost of workaholism and the rewards of recovery.* New York: Harper & Row.

Karasek, R., & Theorell, T. (1990). Healthy work: Stress, productivity, and reconstruction of working life. New York: Basic Books.

Matteson, M. T., & Ivancevich, J. M. (1987). Controlling work stress: Effective human resource and management strategies. San Francisco: Jossey-Bass.

Rosen, R. H. (1991). *The healthy company: Eight strategies to develop people, productivity, and profits.* Los Angeles: Jeremy P. Tarcher.

Schaef, A. W., & Fassel, D. (1988). *The addictive organization.* San Francisco: Harper & Row.

Family Life after Hurricane Andrew: Personal and Phenomenological Reflections

Sherrilyn Coffman

Hurricane Andrew, which devastated the South Florida coast on August 24, 1992, was the most costly natural disaster ever to affect the United States. Over 250,000 persons were left homeless, and multiple health problems were predicted for victims in the months following the hurricane (*Sun-Sentinel*, 1992). On the night of the storm, I sat up with my family, waiting for the full impact to hit my home. But I was one of the fortunate ones; the storm veered and crashed over the coast 50 miles south of us, completely devastating communities in Homestead and South Miami. After it moved out into the Gulf of Mexico, all of us who were South Florida residents, victims and potential victims alike, were left in shock, overwhelmed by the damage. One month later, in

October 1992, I began interviews with 11 families (including 17 children and 13 parents) concerning what it meant to live in South Florida after Hurricane Andrew.

In all phenomenological research, the researcher begins by exploring and recording the personal meaning of the experience being investigated. My own experiences as a potential victim, clinic volunteer, hospital staff nurse, and educator were written in a journal, to help me bracket this information during data collection. This chapter will begin with excerpts from my personal journal, recorded in the days before and after the storm. I will then describe the process of conducting research in this crisis situation. Findings of the phenomenological study, including excerpts from the child and parent interviews, will be presented and discussed.

PERSONAL JOURNALING

The story in my journal begins on Saturday, *August 22,* two days before the hurricane. I was working in the Neonatal Intensive Care Unit at our county hospital. Sometime in the afternoon, I heard other staff talking about a hurricane. It was heading toward South Florida, they said. We had been through this before. Living in this region, each of us had packed our patio furniture and plants into the garage on multiple occasions, only to hear that the hurricane was moving north or south and wouldn't affect us after all. As my shift ended and I left the hospital, I joked with a physician. "I hear that the stores are already sold out. We may starve during this hurricane."

When I woke up the next morning, events started moving much more swiftly. Hurricane Andrew was not only moving our way, but our home was predicted to be in the path of the dangerous storm winds. Now we were forced to consider ourselves potential victims. My husband went out to buy plywood. Lines at hardware stores were already blocks long. Grocery store racks were already empty. For me, peanut butter represented a stockpile that we couldn't live without. None of the grocery stores had any, but we found two small jars at a gasoline station. I felt better. We wouldn't starve.

Off and on during the day before the storm, I was hysterical. My daughter, husband, and I were yelling at one another. We were worried. The urgency of the situation never left us. I remember bursting into tears on more than one occasion. We had friends in the evacuation zone to worry about. How could we help other people when our own preparations were so difficult?

I was so exhausted from the day of preparations, I feel asleep at 11:30 P.M., leaving my husband and daughter to keep watch. I woke at 4 A.M., hearing the rain and wind. Just like a thousand other Florida storms, I thought. Is this hurricane really coming? What I didn't know was that the eye of the storm had taken a path 50 miles south of its predicted range. For most of us in Broward, the county above Miami, our homes were saved, although downed trees and power lines represented a hazard. Our major loss was electricity for a few days. We stayed home and cleaned up the fallen tree limbs in our yards. We listened, glued to the battery-powered radio and TV, as the horrors of Hurricane Andrew were revealed to the world.

The radio and television announcers said, "People's first fear is loss of life. Then property." Property damage took a pale second to the fear of dying. We began to hear the expressions of fear of death from the storm. We heard stories of families moving from room to room in their homes during the course of the storm, to find a location that was still surrounded by walls and a roof. We saw the stunned faces of individuals who had survived in houses totally destroyed by the storm. Many persons commented that this was the closest to death they had ever come. Their horror stories were mixed with thankfulness that they and their family members were still alive.

By the second day, we began to see the photographs of smashed neighborhoods with no buildings left standing; downed trees and power lines; and flooded homes. The hardest hit areas looked like war zones hit by a bomb. Thousands of people were left homeless.

August 26, day 2 after the hurricane: I returned to my job at the College of Nursing today. But I can't get on with my work. The importance of teaching a class can't compare with the disastrous events occurring around me. I pass people on the walk, and they look the same as they did before the hurricane. But when we begin to talk, we share similar feelings. That we have witnessed an event of major proportions. Our exhaustion from fear and worry. Our uncertainty about the outcome of disaster victims. A feeling of helplessness, that we want to help and must help, but don't know how.

August 27, day 3 after the hurricane: Outwardly, life at the college would seem to be going on as usual. But the hurricane seems to have moved inside us, churning up our emotions, attitudes, and lives in general. I said to a fellow faculty member: "It worries me when it starts to feel natural doing all this course preparation. I'm afraid I'll forget that people are hungry and suffering a few miles away." All of us—faculty, students, and staff—are spending a lot of time talking about the meaning of the hurricane.

But I am reaffirming that what I am doing, teaching nursing, *is* important. How else can we give people the skills to respond to a disaster, or to preserve the health of the people affected in this way? We need to think about the long-term effects of what we do, not just the immediate ones. I've seen from the television that even if we canceled school today and all went down to Miami, it would not help. It is chaos down there, and they don't need untrained or disorganized people. Life must go on, and one lesson that I am learning is that life has meaning, even in the mundane, routine things that we do. I am also learning how important everyone is to each other. Garbage collectors and power linemen are some of the most important people in South Florida right now.

August 28, Friday, day 4 after the hurricane: The U.S. Army arrived during the night and already they have set up kitchens to feed the homeless. This was the first day that I saw a disaster victim sobbing during a television interview. Perhaps the adrenalin is wearing off and the reality of the situation is really hitting these people. One of the television reporters commented that there is no one to blame for the damage caused by a hurricane. People are left bewildered about the reasons for their suffering. They can't vent their anger at anyone.

August 29, Saturday, day 5: I went to work at the hospital in South Miami where I am employed part-time. At first sight, the hospital looked intact. However, after a heavy rainstorm later in the day, major roof damage was evident. We had to evacuate patients from several rooms and off units, as water dripped and poured off the ceiling and down walls. The telephone lines didn't always work, and bottled water and sodas had been brought in because the tap water might be contaminated.

About one third of the hospital staff are homeless or have seriously damaged homes. Some have moved in with relatives, and others are living in their dark, hot homes. Each person talked about their damage and where they were during the storm and then said, "But we were lucky." "We didn't lose our roof." "We only had *average* damage." I wonder how long these people can go on this way. They are trying to work, eating meals at the hospital, arranging for care of their children, and cleaning up their homes.

Saturday, *September 5,* day 12: It has been a busy week. I am back to teaching full-time, plus volunteering and working as hospital staff on the weekends. Today I was a nurse volunteer at a newly established clinic in Miami. The clinic is located in a Catholic Church in a neighborhood severely damaged by the hurricane. We saw children and adults in a large, warm room, filled with stacks of medical supplies, tables, and chairs. One patient was a nine-month-old with diarrhea, for whom we prescribed clear fluids and a bland diet. A seven-year-old girl who was complaining of pain in her chest and feeling "nervous" was brought in by her grandmother. She told me, "I think I'm just nervous from the hurricane." Most of the toddlers and school-age children we saw were having physical and emotional reactions, ranging from separation anxiety to depression, minor physical illnesses, psychosomatic symptoms, and fear of rainstorms. Adults' problems ranged from lacerations to "nerves" to exacerbation of chronic illnesses, such as hypertension or diabetes.

THE PHENOMENOLOGICAL STUDY

Because my personal experiences affected me deeply, I felt compelled to document others' perceptions after the disaster. As a pediatric nurse, I was particularly interested in children's and parents' reactions and how recovery from a major natural disaster affected family life. A research proposal was written to explore the experiences of children and parents living in South Florida during the three months following the hurricane. I sought expedited review by our university Human Subjects Committee. Through the assistance of our Dean in the College of Nursing, the study was partially funded by a grant from the Grace Foundation, Boca Raton, Florida.

The purpose of the phenomenological study was to gain a deeper understanding of the nature or meaning of the everyday experiences of children and parents after the natural disaster. The research question explored was: What is the meaning of being a child or parent living in a community affected by a major natural disaster? Hermeneutic phenomenology as described by van Manen (1990) provided the method for the study. Van Manen describes six steps in exploring lived experience: (1) turning to the phenomenon, (2) investigating experience, (3) reflecting on essential themes, (4) writing and rewriting, (5) maintaining focus on the phenomenon, and (6) balancing between parts and the whole.

I had turned inward to the phenomenon through my personal journaling. Investigating experience required that I recruit a purposive sample, so a flyer describing the study was developed and permission was obtained to approach staff at the hospital where I worked part-time. In addition to parents, I specifically sought school-age children (ages 5 through 12). I felt this age group of children would be homogeneous and able to speak to the research question. The final sample was composed of hospital and university staff and their children, as well as other families who were referred by participants. Thirteen parents, including 8 mothers and 5 fathers, and 17 children, including 8 girls and 9 boys, represented 11 families. All participants had lived in the area of the disaster at the time of the storm, but five families had been forced to relocate afterward. In some families, all members were included in the interviews; in other families, only one or a few members were available.

Data collection took place between October and November. The primary source of data was personal interviews. Children were asked to draw pictures. Families also showed me photographs of their destroyed or damaged homes. Field notes were kept during the research process. Additional sources of information were newspaper articles and journal articles.

Interviews took place in homes, offices, a daycare center, and a hospital conference room. All adult participants signed informed consents for themselves and their children before interviews began. Children signed assent forms. Most participants responded eagerly to the research question, "What is it like [to be a parent/to be a kid] after Hurricane Andrew?" Participants were asked to begin by describing an experience related to the research question. They were asked to narrate everything about that experience and other experiences until they had no more to say. Older children and parents used the interviews as opportunities to ventilate and share their feelings and thoughts, often sitting in on family members' interviews to hear each other's impressions. Some of the younger children had more difficulty verbalizing, and needed prompting by their parent or the researcher. When necessary, children were prompted to describe common experiences, such as returning to school. Tape-recorded interviews lasted from 15 minutes to over one hour.

Interviews were transcribed into text and I reflected on lived experiences. Data from children and parents were analyzed separately. Essential themes emerged for each group as I alternated between specific statements and the whole. In general, children described a sense of strangeness, articulated as "life is weird," after the hurricane. Parents' interviews reflected two major themes: (1) parenting was their most important role, and (2) struggles to rebuild family life after the hurricane were superimposed on top of ongoing family issues such as divorce, chronic illness, and adoption.

CHILDREN'S STORIES: "LIFE IS WEIRD"

The 17 children who participated in the study included 8 girls and 9 boys. Ages were distributed as follows: 5 years ($n = 1$), 6 years ($n = 1$), 7 years ($n = 3$), 8 years ($n = 3$), 9 years ($n = 2$), 10 years ($n = 3$), 11 years ($n = 2$), 12 years ($n = 2$). Children were asked to respond to the interview question, "What is it like to be a kid after Hurricane Andrew?" Children responded both verbally and through drawings (Figure 11–1). Each child was assigned a

**Figure 11–1   Alice, Age 6, Drew the Eye of the
Hurricane over a Tree and the Doghouse in Her Backyard**

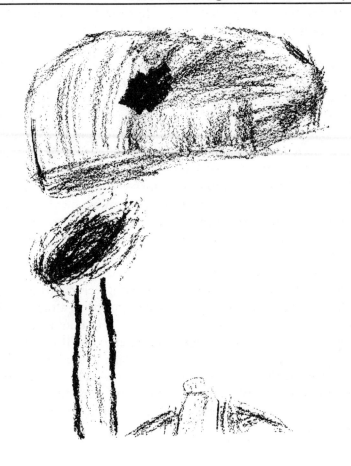

fictitious name during data analysis. Three major themes
emerged from the data analysis of children's interviews: (1) remembering the storm, (2) dealing with the aftereffects, and
(3) reestablishing a life. These major themes and their subthemes
are listed in Table 11-1.

Remembering the Storm

Although the interview question focused on life after the hurricane,
all of the children included events during the storm. Children used

Table 11–1   Themes and Subthemes Identified in Children's Interviews and Drawings

Remembering the Storm

Dealing with the Aftereffects
    Experiencing the Devastation
    Concerns about Safety and Health
    Changes in Relationships

Reestablishing a Life
    Loss of Previous Life-Style
    Constantly Changing
    Experiencing New Things

many descriptive phrases to tell about the sensations they experienced during the hurricane. Ben, age 11, recalled: "It sounded like a train or something was outside. It sounded like all my trees in the back yard were getting ripped out. I was thinking that my house was going to cave in in some parts. I was kind of scared."

Hosea, 9 ½ years old, explained:

And the attic started bumping because of the pressure coming in. And it could have taken the roof off but we all got in the hallway, and the things pounding on the door like football players were trying to break it down.

Maria, 12 years old, described her experience: ". . . suddenly our door started blowing in and out like it was breathing, sort of like cracking. And it was really weird."

Dealing with the Aftereffects

At the time of the interviews, children were still affected by multiple limitations in their daily lives. Their initial reactions to the damage were still vividly remembered, as well as the safety and health hazards posed by environmental changes. Relationships with family and friends were also in flux, and involved experiences of both separation and increased closeness.

Experiencing the Devastation.   Most children described a feeling of shock when they first saw the devastation created in their own neighborhoods. Jason, age 12, described driving home from the hospital where he had stayed with his mother during the storm:

> *When I was riding back there were all these trees and signs messed up, and it was nothing like I'd ever seen before. There was like gas pumps that were real sturdy like flown into the gas stations and like everything was destroyed. All the trees were down and, I don't know, it was a complete mess everywhere.*

The lack of electricity, the unsafe water, and the unsafe conditions both inside and outside their homes left many children bored and tired. Juan, age 10, commented, "I wanted to go outside before the curfew, and I wanted to watch some TV and play little games or something. And I couldn't because I didn't have light or anything."

Talking about their feelings and about the events going on around them was an important activity for these children. Parents, friends, and teachers were most often named as listeners. Lorraine, a fourth grader, commented: "The first day of school we just sat down and everyone talked about where they were and their experience. . . . It gives you a chance to get all your feelings out and express yourself when you go to school." Other children described writing journals and recording interviews of neighbors on tape.

The disaster was also documented through photographs. Melissa, age 7, recalled, "We took pictures of the house with us in front of it." In her drawing of life after the hurricane, Melissa created a detailed picture of her damaged home with herself standing in front, a symbol of life after Hurricane Andrew (Figure 11-2).

Children often expressed gratitude mixed with sadness after the disaster. Melissa remembered, "I was grateful I had a home, and I was glad my cat and my dog survived. My bikes were OK in the shed and trees were down. I was sad about that."

Concerns about Health and Safety.   As described by Gist and Lubin (1989), sleep disorders were mentioned by children and parents as common sequelae to the disaster. Priscilla, 11 years old, remembered a storm that arrived two weeks after the hurricane: ". . . and I kept thinking it was the hurricane and it scared

Figure 11–2 Melissa, Age 7, Represented Life after the Hurricane by Drawing Her Damaged Home with Herself Standing in Front

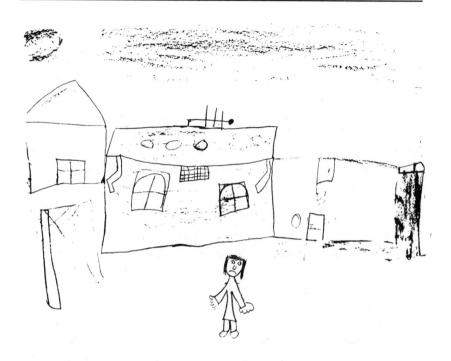

me a lot because it was a storm. And I just couldn't sleep." She also related having a cough from the burning of debris and smoke. Also frequently described, by children of all ages, were nightmares.

Safety concerns were also widespread. Jason, 12 years old, recounted:

I worried about [polluted] water, nails everywhere, big nails and stuff. And I worried about trees coming down, because my brothers and me would go outside in the backyard and swing on the tree branches . . . and the tree could break loose and fall on you.

Juan, age 10, described encountering downed power lines: "Electric wires were in the water, and I crossed one. And I was scared to cross because I couldn't get to the other side because of all those branches."

Changes in Relationships.   Changes in relationships involved growing closer to family members, neighbors, and extended family members. Priscilla described feelings of being closer to her mother and sister. She said, "I got to spend more time with my family. . . . It kind of put us together more as a family."

Many children were taken to stay with relatives during the early weeks after the hurricane, but all children in the study were reunited with their parents by three weeks after the storm. Separation from friends was described as one of the most difficult experiences for these children. Chuck, age 8, talked about what loss of friends meant to his sister: "I felt sad for my sister because all of her friends have been moving away and stuff. And she doesn't have any other friends." Children also mentioned their pets. Johnny, 10 years old, described losing his cat: "We think she committed suicide because she was really weird after the storm. She acted really weird; she acted crazy."

Children described contacts with agencies in the community. Reaching out involved expressing concern and sadness for others less well off after the disaster, as well as accepting help from others. Priscilla related, "A lot of people came up from the church to give us food and stuff, and we were running short of food and water and we didn't have enough money. And everybody kept on saying, 'How was your house?' and you know they treated us real nice."

Reestablishing a Life

For some children, a completely new life-style was required. Those whose families relocated usually had to change schools, make new friends, and adjust to multiple changes. Children who lived in homes that had minimal damage were still greatly affected by the events occurring in the community around them.

Loss of Previous Life-Style.   Susan, age 7 1/2, described losing most of her clothes and toys when her home was destroyed by the storm: "Most of them, they got like blown out the window . . . and they got mold on them, so we only had a few clothes, and those were at Dad's." Older children were especially verbal about the loss they were experiencing. Hosea, 9 1/2 years old, relocated with his family to another county. When asked what was hardest for him to lose, he explained simply:

> *My life. What I do there—everything that I do. How beauti-*
> *ful it was. It was probably one of the most beautiful cities in*
> *the county. I don't think it matters where you live, but*
> *where you grow up is where you want to be.*

Constantly Changing.   The uncertainty that accompanies multiple life changes was often expressed. Susan, in the second grade, described frequent changes at school: "Now it's confusing because we're moving to a different classroom, because there are three classes in there including us. There's one in the morning, and then another class, and then us." Particularly affected by change were children who were forced to relocate. Lorraine, age 9, described what it was like to move to a new apartment:

> *It's different living here because it's a long way from where*
> *we go to school and everything and there isn't much around*
> *here that's the same as our old neighborhood. And I don't*
> *really know anyone around here. I guess it takes getting*
> *used to, but it's just different.*

Experiencing New Things.   Despite the sense of loss, several children described new learning and other gains made since the hurricane. Alice, age 6, described making new friends in her neighborhood: "It's fun, because I get to see my friends a lot. And I like to have new friends and now I have a lot of new friends." Hosea, a fourth grader, described watching news broadcasts on television and reading the newspaper to learn more about the hurricane. Another child described working harder on homework, because she couldn't play as much after school. Priscilla, age 11, described lessons she had learned for the future:

> *I think it is better to go through the hurricane as a child than as an adult. Because when you're a child, and you grow up, you might have to do it again. I'd rather go through it as a child and know what to do when I'm an adult and have kids.*

PARENTS' STRUGGLES TO REBUILD FAMILY LIFE

Eight mothers and five fathers were also interviewed for the study. Parents responded to the interview question, "What is it like to be a parent after Hurricane Andrew?" Two major themes were expressed in the parent interviews: (1) parenting was seen by these individuals as their most important role, and (2) struggles to rebuild family life after the hurricane were superimposed on top of ongoing family issues such as divorce, chronic illness, unemployment, and adoption. Major themes and subthemes are listed in Table 11-2.

Parenting: The Most Important Role

Parents emphatically noted the importance of their roles as parents. One mother began her interview by stating, "Being a parent is the most important role in my life . . . and especially during and

Table 11–2　Themes and Subthemes Identified in Parents' Interviews

Major Themes
　Parenting: The Most Important Role
　On Top of Everything Else
　　Overwhelmed by Damage and Demands
　　Thankful for What We Have
　　Limited by Aftereffects
　　Responsible for Family
　　Balancing Roles and Needs
　　Constantly Changing Amid Uncertainty
　　Finding Meaning and Growing Stronger

after the hurricane." Decisions about their children's well-being predominated in the first days and weeks after the storm; they ranged from immediately checking on children from whom they were separated during the storm, to arranging for their safety during the clean-up process. One father, who fearfully waited through the hurricane alone, described emerging from the house after the storm: "I immediately thought about . . . the kids and tried to call." A mother summarized her view of parenting after the hurricane: "It's made the whole experience harder, because [the children] have always been first and foremost in our lives and in our minds—my husband and I both."

On Top of Everything Else

A phrase spoken by several of the parents was: "on top of" or "on top of everything else." This phrase had several different meanings in the study: (1) parenting was the *topmost role* described by parents; (2) problems created by the hurricane were imposed *on top of* ongoing family issues (adoption, job responsibilities, marriage); and (3) parents often identified a *hierarchy of needs* (like Maslow's pyramid) beginning with a focus on survival during the storm, advancing to concerns for safety, food, and medical care, and ending with references to spirituality and clarification of values.

Feeling secure that his wife and children were safe at the hospital where his wife worked during the storm, one father described his personal struggle: "Once the house started being damaged pretty severely, I forgot about everything except self-preservation; I really very nearly panicked at a time when the electricity went out and several windows broke at the same time. I just prayed like I never prayed before with my face in the floor."

The demands of parenting were superimposed on top of job demands. Strained to the breaking point, these parents were also nurses, teachers, police officers, and firefighters. One woman described the demands of her supervisory position: "It was hard because when you're in charge everyone looks up to you for guidance. It's very hard to give to other people when you're hurting too."

Major life changes, such as marriage and adoption, gave a special meaning to the difficulties created by the hurricane. The adopting mother of an infant whose adoption proceedings had not been finalized described her fears: "And we were afraid because we lost our home, the adoption wouldn't be finalized. And they assured us it would, because it was just an unusual situation. But it was kind of scary." A new parent, who had been married just the year before, described the buildup of events: "And it was just like one more added thing. I was handling the parent thing pretty well, but when it came to the rest of it, it was the culmination. And it has put a lot of stress between [my wife] and I."

Overwhelmed by Damage and Demands.   Tremendous difficulties in all activities of daily living resulted from the damage to the environment caused by the rain and winds. One parent described the damage to her apartment complex: "Half the apartments in our building were uninhabitable. The building stretches north and south and all of the windows facing east were blown in by the winds. The roof of the building was lifted off—just gone. You could stand in the living room of one of those east-facing apartments and look at the sky. There had been people living in those apartments when the storm hit, and they were stumbling around outside, numb, weeping. It was like being in a war." This parent further described the effects of the storm:

> *When we moved here, this was a lush and verdant place. We were surrounded by mature trees. We had a giant canopy of foliage outside our windows which offered beauty and privacy and quiet, and it is gone now. . . . It is going to be years and years before the beauty of the surroundings is restored, if ever.*

Many parents described special ways of coping with the disaster. One mother commented: "It took me a few days. I pretty much stayed in the first few days, because we couldn't even stand to go out the front door or back door and look at all the other destruction. I could only handle what had been destroyed at my house."

Thankful for What We Have.   The families who participated in the study were fortunate that no members were injured during the storm, but several families lost their homes. Descriptions of shock were followed by expressions of joy among many parents. One father focused on an "overwhelming joy to be alive," despite severe damage to his home. A more fortunate parent described returning to her house after the storm: "When I saw my house, I walked around and the walls were OK and the windows were OK and the glass was OK. I couldn't believe it. The relief. I just couldn't believe it. And I really thought that God has really helped me and protected me. It was like a bubble was over my house. I was so thankful."

Limited by Aftereffects.   Major environmental limitations affected all families, even those whose homes were intact: "It was mind-boggling. We had no power. We had a portable radio that we were trying to play only at intervals. Using candles to light the house and trying not to open the refrigerator." There were other types of limitations, also. One mother commented: "I have a lot of days when I have to tell people, I can't think about that today. As soon as I am able to think about that, or deal with it, I will let you know. And it is terrible, but the alternative is pretending that you are capable, when you are not."

Responsible for Family.   The responsibilities of parenting were described as the most important factors in the participants' decision making after the hurricane: "There was no choice involved; there were other people to think about, besides just ourselves. Part of our big rush to try to find a place as quickly as we did was so that [the children] could get settled and mainly so that they could start school on time."

Safety concerns were prominent because of major environmental hazards: exposed swimming pools, broken tiles, nails, and piles of trash. The mother of three small children focused on these issues: "My big concern was keeping the kids safe. And even though I didn't worry about them getting outside of the house, it was just as dangerous inside the house with broken glass everywhere. It was just a complete safety hazard."

Balancing Roles and Needs.   Most parents found it impossible to care for their children and deal with severely damaged homes in the first few days after the storm. Friends or relatives outside the disaster area were asked to provide child care. One parent who lost her home described her situation: "A few days after the hurricane, I decided to take the kids up north to be with the grandparents. . . . I wanted them to be able to be around people who could talk to them more and interact with them more, and I couldn't. I was emotionally drained myself; I really couldn't do it. I felt like I wasn't able to be a real good parent at that time after the hurricane, because I was too preoccupied with a million and one other things."

Constantly Changing Amid Uncertainty.   As in the children's interviews, multiple life changes were described by parents. One father described a new philosophy in his reaction to change: "What I'm looking forward to is to be able to grow and deal with changes that I'm going to experience, because I know that they're going to be coming. I just want to be in a situation where I feel I'm on my feet, and I can deal with the change. It was difficult in that I didn't feel like I was on solid ground."

Because of multiple changes, one mother described her efforts to maintain the same school for her children: "We thought it was one thing we could keep the same for them because they had been through so many changes—the separation, then the hurricane. We'd been burglarized just before the hurricane, so it was just one thing after the other."

Finding Meaning and Growing Stronger.   All of the parents reaffirmed the importance of the family and their roles as parents. Parents actively searched for meaning in the disaster, and described how their values had changed as a result of their experiences. These statements took various forms, according to each individual's life situation.

One mother commented: "I feel totally different about possessions than I used to. I now feel like giving up all possessions and taking a vow of poverty, which is all I've got. I just feel like I want to be done with all the disappointment that comes from physical things. I could be happy with fewer dresses, less furniture, fewer dinners out, and more time, because time is a lot of what determines the quality of our lives, I think."

A father described efforts to teach his children important lessons about life: "We chose early on to try to teach the kids a lesson or to set an example of a survivor. We felt that was very important. We didn't want them to be around people who were victims. We wanted them to be around people who were survivors, who were taking a positive approach to pulling themselves out of the storm."

DISCUSSION

The significance of profound environmental changes is vividly portrayed in the descriptions of these children and parents. There is no doubt that the hurricane's aftereffects created havoc in the lives of these families. Parents described difficulties in carrying out daily tasks, making decisions, supporting their children, and maintaining marital relationships. Children described fears of injury and storm recurrence, constant change in school and family routines, and loss of friends. However, in creating meaning out of the disaster, both parents and children described ways in which events after the hurricane had helped them to recognize and utilize their strengths.

All South Florida residents were deeply affected by the widespread damage from the storm. Even those of us who were potential victims felt the aftereffects, as we watched our friends and coworkers struggling, and participated in the recovery effort. To various extents, each of us was challenged to create meaning from the disaster, and to clarify our own values and priorities.

A review of literature on families' reactions after natural disaster revealed little descriptive material about everyday experiences of children and parents in that situation. The literature did focus on symptomatology, and participants in this study described many of the symptoms listed as expected emotional reactions to disaster. For adults, these included disbelief, a sense that life was out of balance, sadness, anger, impaired concentration, and a desire to get "back to normal" (Stanley, 1990). For children, reactions included sleep disorders, excessive fears, and persistent anxiety (Farberow & Frederick, 1978; Gist & Lubin, 1989). But the rich descriptions of parents and children in this study went beyond symptomatology. Their comments also reflected altruism, responsibility for others, renewed spirituality, and clarification of values that reflected strength and growth after the crisis. Many of these same behaviors were found in the victims of the earlier Hurricane Hugo in South Carolina (Weinrich, Hardin, & Johnson, 1990). These reactions provide validity for the basic assumption of most community treatment programs after major disasters: disaster victims are normal people encountering abnormal circumstances. Therefore, interventions for families should be planned not only to compensate for deficits, but also to build on strengths and reaffirm them.

As residents of South Florida recovering from Hurricane Andrew, we have learned that Mother Nature can be violent and destructive. Our lives can be turned upside-down overnight, resulting in chaos and confusion. Some of us have lost homes; others, our way of life. We have shared in each other's suffering and wept together. But we have also learned that we are capable of helping each other, of overcoming difficulties, and of working together in seemingly impossible situations. We have seen the importance of each person in a family or in a community, and have come to better appreciate each person's contribution. Through confronting our own mortality, each of us has been challenged to reconsider our values and reformulate our possible futures. Thus, Mother Nature is also a teacher who provides important lessons for each of us.

PERSONAL STATEMENT

I've always been a "people" person. I tolerated pets. I decided to recycle because it benefited people. I went into nursing because I wanted to help people. As a pediatric nurse, I was attracted to children and families who had serious, devastating problems. I became a clinical specialist with children with myelomeningocele and spinal cord injuries. I felt that these children and parents had the greatest needs, and I could do something to help.

I loved the outdoors because it had given me so much pleasure as a kid. I grew up in rural southern Indiana, where my favorite place to play was the woods across the road, and I visited my grandparents' farm every summer. I took nature's beauty for granted, because it had been a regular part of my life. Even as an adult, I didn't take the environment seriously; I viewed it as the background against which people's needs predominated.

Years later, when Hurricane Andrew struck South Florida, I was stunned! I found myself in the midst of a situation where nature's forces had destroyed people's homes, life-styles, and lives. The environment demanded my attention in a way that it never had before. Although only a potential victim, I was glued to the television set, observing how survivors in the disaster zone reacted to the total devastation. My natural reaction was to want to help the people involved. As a researcher, I felt that documenting people's experiences would help us gain something from the disaster.

But I have gained more than research findings. From my experiences after the hurricane, I have come to appreciate how dependent we are on our natural environment. We take for granted the usual balance between people and nature. When events such as Hurricane Andrew occur, we are reminded of the awesome power of nature and our complete dependence on it. From my studies of family members' reactions after the hurricane, I have also come to appreciate our resilience as humans, our ability to overcome disaster, and our openness to learning the lessons that nature teaches.

REFERENCES

Farberow, N., & Frederick, C. (1978). *Training manual for human service workers in major disasters.* DHHS Publication No. (ADM) 90-538. Washington, DC: Government Printing Office.

Gist, R., & Lubin, B. (1989). *Psychosocial aspects of disaster.* New York: John Wiley & Sons.

Stanley, S. (1990). When the disaster is over: Helping the healers to mend. *Journal of Psychosocial Nursing, 28*(5), 12–16.

Sun-Sentinel. (1992). *Andrew! Savagery from the sea.* Orlando, FL: Tribune Publishing.

van Manen, M. (1990). *Researching lived experience.* New York: SUNY Press.

Weinrich, S., Hardin, S., & Johnson, M. (1990). Nurses respond to Hurricane Hugo victims' disaster stress. *Archives of Psychiatric Nursing, 4*(3), 195–205.

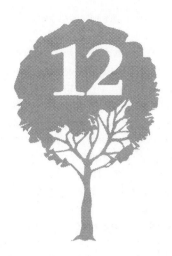

Emotional and Environmental Connections: Impact of the Armenian Earthquake

Anie Sanentz Kalayjian

INTRODUCTION

As environmental disasters occur with increasing frequency, their impact also grows more severe. There are two kinds of environmental disasters: (1) man-made or "human-induced" and (2) natural. Natural disasters are referred to as acts of "Mother Nature" or "acts of God." They constitute a category of environmental events that periodically subject human systems to a wide range of disruptions and increased stress (Bolin, 1989). Man-made or human-induced environmental disasters include most energy-industry or related accidents, such as fires, coal mine and natural gas explosions, hydroelectric dam failures, and nuclear plant malfunctions. Between 1944 and 1987, there were 284 nuclear accidents worldwide, many of which were caused, at least in part, by the mishandling of isotopes or inadvertent exposure to X-rays (United Nations Environment Program, 1993–1994).

Trends of the past two decades suggest that both the frequency and the magnitude of natural disasters may continue to increase at a rapid rate. It has been estimated that, over the past 20 years, natural disasters claimed over three million lives, and adversely affected another one billion. Although natural disasters are estimated to claim an average of 25,000 lives per year (IE/PAC, 1992), in 1988, the Armenian earthquake alone resulted in over 25,000 deaths. The United Nations General Assembly adopted a resolution declaring the 1990s the International Decade for Natural Disaster Reduction, and the U.S. Senate and House of Representatives endorsed the Decade concept in resolutions passed the following year. The National Committee for the International Decade for Natural Disaster Reduction (IDNDR) was formed to provide encouragement to government agencies, as well as private groups and individuals, to be involved in relevant disaster reduction activities.

In my capacity as the World Federation for Mental Health representative at the United Nations, I was fortunate to take part in a special conference on mental health, at which I presented my research findings on the psychosocial impact of natural disasters. This chapter includes segments from that presentation.

During the past decade, devastating earthquakes have struck in California (Coalinga, San Francisco, and the San Fernando Valley), Idaho, West Africa, Belgium, Turkey, Japan, the Philippines, Hawaii, Armenia, Georgia, India, Mexico, Indonesia, and Peru. Other natural disasters—such as severe flooding in the Mississippi region of the United States, in Bangladesh, and in Pakistan; brush fires in California and Spain; typhoons and tsunamis (tidal waves) in Japan; hurricanes in South Carolina and Southern Florida; volcanic activity in the Pacific Rim, particularly in the Philippines— also have occurred within the past ten years.

Natural disasters are unavoidable; no region or country is immune. Scientists agree that one cannot stop natural disasters from happening. What we can do, and must do, is (1) work on reducing their impact via education and training, and (2) increase and perfect the warning and prediction systems through research and technological advancement.

This chapter focuses on the impact of a particular natural disaster—the earthquake in Armenia—and explores the survivors' meanings of emotional and environmental connectedness. The conceptual framework comprises Gaian principles of ecology and Franklinian logotherapeutic and existential perspectives, couched in the frameworks of posttraumatic stress disorder (PTSD) and nursing process. First, these perspectives are briefly reviewed. The chapter then emphasizes the psychosocial response of Armenian survivors to the earthquake. The social responses to natural disaster are called "secondary stresses"; they expose victims to long-term, response-generated demands (Quarantelli, 1985) He distinguished between disaster-produced stress and response-generated demands in order to determine types and extent of mental health services needed in the aftermath.

The utilization of the nursing process in developing and managing the Mental Health Outreach Program (MHOP) for Armenia—which I cofounded immediately after the earthquake—is also demonstrated. The chapter concludes with a brief review of the post-natural-disaster therapeutic interventions utilized with survivors in Armenia. These same interactions later proved effective in helping survivors in Southern Florida and Southern California.

CONCEPTUAL FRAMEWORK

Frankl's Logotherapeutic and Existential Perspectives

According to Frankl (1978), being human is being always directed and pointed to something or someone other than oneself—to a meaning to fulfill, or another human being to encounter, or a cause to serve, or a person to love. Only to the extent that one is living out this self-transcendence of human existence is one truly human or does one become one's true self.

Each life situation is unique; therefore, the meaning of each situation must be unique (Frankl, 1978). As Frankl called the suffering man the homo patients, I called the quake survivors the homo survivors. I was impressed by their ability to suffer and yet to mold their suffering into a human achievement, with a new meaning and a connectedness with self, others, and the Earth.

Just as people differ in their perceptions of trauma and in the ways they cope with it, they also differ in the meanings attributed to the same situation (Frankl, 1969). Frankl focused on the uniqueness of meanings, in terms of both essence and existence. According to Christou (1976), meaning in psychology refers to the experiencing soul and must be clearly differentiated from meaning as it relates to thought and thought processes, and from meaning as it is attached to sense perception. In defining psychotherapy, Christou underscored the significance of a "logos of the soul"— the meaning of life and the meaning and value of one's own psychological experience.

Two other theorists have expressed ideas on meaning. Carl Jung (1972) stated that finding meaning in life was a difficult task, and he believed that most of us are not forced to answer this fatal question of the meaning of life. Alfred Adler (1932/1980) stated that every human being had a meaning of life by the age of five, and that this meaning—although unconscious—objectively existed.

Frankl (1984) maintained that, so long as we are breathing, our life has meaning—whether we believe it or not, whether we have discovered it or not, whether we admit it or not. Leo Tolstoy, in his book *My Confession,* reinforced Frankl's assertion that life has meaning and that we must have the mental capacity to understand it (Leontiev, 1992).

I believe that all children develop unique and distinctive sets of meanings. These meanings remain unconscious until an extraordinary event forces them up to a conscious and more accessible level. Furthermore, the meanings are dynamic—always changing and developing to meet existential and spiritual needs.

GAIAN AND ECOLOGICAL PERSPECTIVES

Gaia, also spelled Gaea, or simply G—the Greek word for Earth— has always been deemed feminine. *She* is Mother Earth; the provider of all sustenance; the fertile soil that supplies the food we eat, the tools we need, the air we breathe, and the water we drink. The image of Gaia through the centuries—even before humans began formal recording—was one of a living, female entity (Allaby, 1989).

The Gaian image of Earth, first proposed by Lovelock (1979) some twenty years ago, is of a living supersystem. To Lovelock, the Gaia hypothesis is an alternative to the pessimistic view of nature as a primitive force to be subdued and conquered. According to Allaby (1989), who has worked closely with Lovelock for many years, a system is an entity distinguishable from all other systems; it is a single, living entity that responds appropriately to changes. Thus, within this living superorganism, each animal and plant serves a specific function, thereby maintaining a stable, living whole. Each animal and plant can also cause severe damage by disturbing the Earth's regulatory mechanisms, especially when interfering with the climate.

There are many examples of how our behavior causes damage to the Earth. Noteworthy here are: the greenhouse effect, global warming or cooling, and a decrease in the levels of carbon dioxide. When life began on Earth, carbon dioxide accounted for about 30% of the volume of the atmosphere (300,000 parts of carbon dioxide to every million parts of the total atmosphere). Today, the air contains only 0.03% carbon dioxide (about 300 parts per million). According to Allaby (1989), if this trend continues to where the concentration is reduced to about half its present level, or around 150 parts per million, most plants would die. The climate was regulated for a billion years by living organisms. This was achieved through the removal of carbon dioxide from the atmosphere and the secure long-term storage of the carbon dioxide to produce the opposite of a greenhouse effect. Therefore, fluctuations in carbon dioxide will ultimately cause fluctuations in the climate. Volcanoes would continue to release carbon dioxide and, with the rate of biological removal reduced, it would add to the accumulation. This accumulation will ultimately cause a failure in the Earth's self-regulatory process. As Lovelock (1979) asserted, the atmospheric concentration of gases such as oxygen and ammonia is found to be kept at an optimum value from which even small departures could have disastrous consequences for life.

Human beings—among the many animals on Earth—have often disregarded the laws of Nature, to their own disadvantage. Goldsmith (1993) cited Richard St. Barbe-Baker's profound assertion that, almost everywhere, humans have rampaged over the earth, forgetting that they are only one of the players put here to play a part in harmony and oneness with all other living things. According to Valdov (1993), humans have done this because they have a significant gift for denial. In my opinion, although we have done this overtly in the name of technological advancement and scientific pursuit, covertly we have been driven by thanatos—the death instinct.

Ludwig von Bertalanffy (1970), a systems theorist, said that living systems display qualities that are not apparent when studying the systems' parts, but only become apparent once we see a system as a whole. This is congruent with the writings of Goldsmith (1993), in that the coordination of the behavior of the parts by the whole is only apparent once one identifies the whole. That parts of a living system cooperate not just with each other but with the whole, and that they are homeotelic—seeking order and stability—has been reinforced by many holistic nursing theorists.

To maintain a healthy environmental status, as well as a healthy emotional and physical status, we need to communicate, cooperate, and collaborate. As Odum asserts, humanity needs to emulate cooperation for mutual benefit—a survival strategy that is quite common in natural systems (Goldsmith, 1993).

EARTHQUAKE IN ARMENIA

On December 7, 1988, a massive earthquake shook Soviet Armenia—presently the Republic of Armenia—measuring 6.8 on the Richter scale. The earthquake occurred in an area highly vulnerable to seismic activity. It destroyed two-thirds of Leninakan (population 300,000), half of Kirovakan (population 150,000), totally destroyed Spitak (a town of about 30,000, situated at the epicenter of the quake), and leveled some 56 villages. In the end, the official death toll had reached 25,000, and 500,000 others were handicapped, homeless, or otherwise affected (Kalayjian, 1994a).

During the ten months preceding the earthquake, Armenia was in the throes of a sociopolitically tense and economically drained climate, because of a conflict with neighboring Azerbaijan over Nagorno-Karabagh, a 4,000-square-kilometer enclave mostly populated by Armenians and locally ruled by Armenians until 1923, when Joseph Stalin gave this area to Soviet Azerbaijan. In early 1988, with the emergence of *glasnost* and *perestroika,* Armenia challenged Soviet Premier Mikhail Gorbachev by testing the new attempts at democracy. As a result, over 300,000 Armenian refugees from Azerbaijan came to already crowded Armenia. In February 1988, there were pogroms in Sumgait, Azerbaijan, where dozens of Armenians were killed, houses were burned, and women were raped and set on fire (Kalayjian, 1991).

Noteworthy here is the parallel between the seismologists' description of the quake area—as a structural knot, engendered by the interaction of several rigid plates (Sullivan, 1988)—and the sociopolitical and emotional status of the region—political agitation, tension, anger, resentment, disappointment, and mistrust, due to rigid attitudes.

POSTTRAUMATIC STRESS DISORDER

The term posttraumatic stress disorder (PTSD) was coined in the early 1970s when addressing the psychosocial needs of Vietnam veterans returning home to America. Previously called "shell shock" or "combat fatigue," PTSD attempted to describe these unique needs of these individuals after experiencing disasters.

According to the American Psychiatric Association's *Diagnostic and Statistical Manual of Mental Disorders,* Fourth Edition (DSM-IV), published in 1994, PTSD is defined as the development of characteristic symptoms following an extreme traumatic stressor involving direct personal experience of an event that involves actual or threatened death or injury, or a threat to the physical integrity of self, a family member, or another close associate (Criterion A1); the presence of intense fear, helplessness, or horror (Criterion A2); characteristic symptoms, including the persistent reexperiencing of the traumatic incident (Criterion B);

persistent avoidance of stimuli or numbing of general responsiveness (Criterion C); and persistent increased arousal (Criterion D). These symptoms must be present for more than one month (Criterion E), and the disturbance must cause impairment in social, occupational, emotional, or other areas of functioning (Criterion F).

The following are some examples of traumatic events: military combat, violent personal assault, tortures, natural or human-induced disasters, environmental accidents, severe automobile accidents, chronic fatal illnesses, and similar occurrences.

MENTAL HEALTH OUTREACH PROGRAM

Immediately after the earthquake, I went to Armenia to assess the mental health needs of the survivors, which became the first formal step of the Mental Health Outreach Program (MHOP) for Armenia. The nursing process included assessment, diagnosis, planning, implementation, and evaluation (Alfaro, 1986). For the purposes of MHOP, I expanded the nursing process from these original five phases into eight phases. The use of this expanded version of the nursing process to develop post-natural-disaster outreach programs, nationally and internationally, has been a challenging and rewarding experience. These are the eight phases of the post-natural-disaster Mental Health Outreach Program (MHOP):

1. Preassessment;
2. Assessment;
3. Analysis;
4. Community diagnoses;
5. Planning;
6. Implementation;
7. Evaluation;
8. Remodification

Based on the on-site assessment, a short-term, six-month plan was developed to address the mental health needs of the survivor community (Kalayjian, 1994b).

RESEARCH STUDY

Sample

Four to six weeks after the earthquake, I interviewed survivors at five shelters located in Soviet Armenia, until the desired sample size (N = 60) was reached. Survivors ranged from 22 to 65 years in age, with a majority (75%) being between the ages of 30 and 60. Half of all respondents were male. A majority (68%) were college-educated. Over 62% were married. The overwhelming majority (98%) had lost their jobs as a result of the earthquake, and had been forced to relocate. All had incurred physical and monetary losses.

Instrument

I reviewed many posttraumatic stress disorder (PTSD) assessment instruments for their applicability. The clarity and brevity of the Reaction Index Scale (Frederick, 1986) made it the instrument of choice for me, given a chaotic disaster milieu in which expeditious assessment was a requisite for the effective implementation of the Mental Health Outreach Program in Armenia. This 28-item instrument for adults (20 items for children) has a scoring range of 0 to 4 for each item, with a total of 80 possible points. Scoring is bidirectional. Both parts of the instrument (adult and child) were translated into Eastern Armenian, the language of the survivor community. (Encouraged by the effectiveness of this instrument, I used it again in the subsequent disasters in Southern Florida and Southern California.)

A variety of other instruments were utilized with children and adolescents, based on their age, emotional readiness, and level of understanding. Structured and unstructured drawings were utilized to assess the level of trauma in children under the age of 10. A structured drawing is one in which the child is given specific directions as to what to draw. Adolescents were given sentence completions, as well as the Reaction Index Scale.

In this chapter, I will focus on adult survivors' responses.

Results

A majority of respondents (78%) scored higher than 50% on the Reaction Index Scale, indicating severe levels of posttraumatic stress disorder (PTSD). Fear was the most frequently expressed difficulty (F = 98). "I am really scared; I try not to think about it [the quake], but it is still in front of my eyes." "No one should endure this much suffering and pain." "If they had told me that there was a horror movie such as this [the quake], I would not have believed it."

Most of the respondents (F = 50) expressed fear coupled with feelings of uncertainty pertaining to their connectedness to the Earth, to "Motherland." Violent aftershocks had continued for two months following the initial quake, and, with each aftershock, the sense of uncertainty had been exacerbated. Every bulldozer or truck passing by and causing a minor tremor would jolt the people, disconnecting them from their beliefs regarding the environment and the "Mother Earth," the "Holy Earth." "This is the land of our great-great-greatgrandparents; our roots are here." "We have been here [in the general region of Asia Minor and the Caucasus] for over three millennia, we're not going to leave no matter what," expressed many others heroically.

Other uncertainties caused by the quake overwhelmed many respondents: "What's going to happen to our house?" "Are they [the government] going to provide us with food?" "Are they going to rebuild our houses?" asked others, focusing on their basic needs for shelter and food. Some survivors were more pessimistic and fatalistic in their expressions: "Nothing is certain when the earth itself moves under your feet," and "If this quake could destroy our country in forty seconds, what is the use of all the planning we do in life—all for nothing!"

Uncertainty coupled with fear overwhelmed survivors and influenced all aspects of their lives, as well as their decision making. They feared the death of loved ones (62%); therefore, they indicated behaving more protectively (58%). They expressed feelings of helplessness and hopelessness (50%). Some survivors expressed anger toward God or the Creator (11%), and, of these, 56% felt guilty for expressing such anger, for this challenged their religious beliefs. Of those respondents with children (N = 32), a majority (98%) stated that the behavior of their children had changed. Some of these changes were: bed wetting, insomnia, attention deficit, withdrawal, and verbal and physical aggression.

Anger was expressed very frequently (F = 90). Anger was expressed toward others: the Azeris and the Turks (87%), the Soviet regime (85%), the builders and the engineers (83%), the Soviet Armenian caregivers and "doctors" (80%), the Soviet Government (76%), "our bad luck and fate" (70%), and God (11%).

Anger at oneself was also expressed, in the form of feelings of guilt. There was guilt for surviving (61%): "They're lucky and fortunate [those who died]"; guilt for not being able to rescue a loved one (28%): "I could hear him yelling for help, and I couldn't do anything about it, I can still hear him"; and guilt for expressing anger toward the Creator (6%). Anger toward the deceased was not expressed. Survivors talked about the deceased as being perfect: "He was the smartest, top of his class," or "She was the most beautiful girl in Spitak, kind, caring and sensitive, a living saint."

Some survivors (38%) expressed feelings of emptiness, frustration, and apathy. A majority of respondents (92%) admitted to having violent nightmares about the earthquake. The themes of nightmares usually corresponded to the feelings expressed earlier by these respondents. In their nightmares, dead relatives and loved ones were haunting them, and pulling or calling them; the quake was recurring and their lives were in danger; houses were burning and survivors were dying. Some survivors (11%) expressed feeling more and more disconnected from their "Motherland." Those survivors expressed plans to leave Armenia as soon as possible, disappointment, and disconnection.

When asked about the meaning of the earthquake, a majority of survivors (78%) called it "fate," "kismet," or "bad luck." Respondents repeatedly mentioned the Ottoman Turkish Genocide of the Armenians in 1915, and the Sumgait massacre of 1988, as proof that calamities repeatedly befell Armenians. "Why us? Why the Armenians? We're but a handful," and "What have we done to the Almighty to deserve this?" many respondents exclaimed helplessly. These respondents had high scores on the Reaction Index Scale, indicating severe levels of PTSD.

One in five survivors interviewed (20%) had positive value and meaning orientation referring to the earthquake. They attributed meaning to reaching beyond themselves, volunteering to work with and help other survivors. They revealed that caring and ministering to others, helping one another, were the real meanings they had attributed to the quake. They not only expressed having valued what they had learned from their experiences, but used this insight to help other survivors. The above respondents also found meaning through acceptance of what was beyond their control: "We could not have prevented it [the quake]." They then went on to modify their attitudes: "I am changing the way I look at things; although I've lost everything, everything material, I have myself and I have this moment with you on this Earth; no one or no situation can take that away from me," and "We live in a mountainous region, where seismic activity is not uncommon. If you read our history, you'll notice that a devastating quake had struck this area some one hundred years ago; we rebuilt then and we'll do the same now—even better!" They also reiterated convictions such as: "I am stronger now," "We [the Armenians] are an indomitable nation; we dealt with the Ottoman Turkish Genocide when over two million Armenians were killed; we dealt with the seventy years of Stalinist regime, losing many more lives; we dealt with the Azeris, yet losing more lives—and now we deal with this devastating quake and the Azeri blockade of food. We can deal with anything!"

The remaining 2% were in the process of finding a meaning.

Discussion

According to Frankl (1969), suffering becomes meaningful as one takes a stand toward it, showing an ability to self-transcend, to detach oneself from one's predicament and to change one's attitude. This is how one can accept fate and add deeper meaning to one's own life.

Uncertainty.   Uncertainty was the most frequently expressed coping difficulty. In a previous study that I had conducted with spouses of cancer patients, uncertainty was also one of the major coping difficulties expressed (Kalayjian, 1989). The spouses' uncertainty was qualitatively different from the quake survivors' in that it referred to more emotional uncertainties of self, to death and dying, and to challenged feelings of immortality—all unrelated to the environment or the Earth.

Meaning. Those earthquake survivors who were able to find meaning in their situation (20%) were able to achieve this meaning through what Frankl (1986) has called "dereflection," to counteract the feelings of "hyperreflection." Dereflection means turning one's attention away from self and one's own particular situation. According to Goldsmith (1993), this type of behavior requires the involvement of our instincts, emotions, and values, which must be mediated at the primitive level. He further stated that our most fundamental knowledge of our relationship with the world around us falls into this category of knowing, which he also called "intuition." Indeed, Goldsmith (1993) continued, if our society and the Gaian hierarchy are to maintain their stability or continuity, then this fundamental knowledge must be transmitted intact from one generation to the next.

Intuition. Many female survivors expressed feeling "like something very tragic was going to happen." "I felt very sad, I couldn't explain it." Those mothers who had newborn infants described how their babies saved them: "My baby was crying at the top of her lungs; so I had to leave my house, to take her outside; and the earthquake struck, my house was demolished, but we were fine." "My mother was babysitting; I was working; my baby was crying so much; my mother called me to come home from the factory to take her to the doctor. I left the factory, and the earthquake happened. All my coworkers are dead, except me; my baby saved me." Although intuition has been challenged by modern-day scientists, it is also considered a "seventh sense," a "supreme wisdom" that cannot be acquired in universities or institutions of higher education. We, as nurses—predominantly female professionals—have been identified as possessing this kind of knowledge, and for the past few decades we have attempted to establish a scientific basis for it.

From my experience working with natural disasters, I have found that animals have been the first to flee the area before an earthquake. Many anecdotal stories of the survivors in Armenia and California reinforced my observation that animals have increased connectedness with the Earth. Furthermore, the alleged ability of so-called "earthquake-sensitive" persons to predict earthquakes is worthy of scientific exploration.

Anger. Anger was expressed very frequently. This is contrary to previous research in this area, where natural disasters are referred to as "acts of God," a label that automatically eliminates human involvement and leaves no target of resentment and anger (Sorensen et al., 1987). Thus, the Azeris, the Turks, the Soviet regime, the Soviet authorities, the Soviet caregivers, the builders, Fate, and God were all targeted.

Anger toward the deceased was suppressed, because this is socially unacceptable. Instead, survivors placed the deceased on a pedestal. Deceased boys were described as "smart," "brilliant," "top of his class"; and deceased girls as "beautiful," "sensitive," "kind," and "saintly." This is indicative of cultural, gender-specific values. Anger toward the deceased was displaced onto other survivors—siblings, friends, and neighbors. As Levinson (1989) pointed out, the deceased are usually stripped of their human and sometimes imperfect qualities, thus inhibiting the grief process.

Denial. The findings of my study also revealed the presence of denial as defined by Kubler-Ross (1969). Survivors went through a phase of emotionally refusing to believe that death had occurred. They expressed a wish to bargain to exchange places with the dead, and refused to dispose of the belongings of the deceased. Because many bodies were buried in the rubble, burned, or just not found, this denial phase was extended. Eight weeks after the quake, survivors were still looking for their family members, friends, and coworkers.

According to Fabry (1980), repressed traumas can cause neuroses; ignored meanings can cause emptiness, frustration, value conflicts, and depression. The findings of my study reinforced these assertions, in that a majority (78%) of those who expressed meaninglessness also expressed feelings of emptiness, frustration, and value conflict, which was a basis for their depression, severe levels of PTSD, and existential frustration.

At the World Congress of Logotherapy in 1989, Frankl, responding to my question, asserted that fulfillment of inner meaning is relatively independent of external circumstances; it can be achieved even in adverse circumstances; and the search for meaning is relatively independent of external circumstances. The findings of this study were congruent with this notion: 20% of respondents expressed positive value and meaningful orientation.

Meaning in Suffering.   According to Frankl (1969), it is part of human nature, especially one's spirit, to reach beyond the self, to make use of one's own capacity for self-transcendence, to forget the self, and to help others. Although almost all respondents stated that they had helped one another, only 20% attributed meaning to this behavior. Thus, only one in five respondents perceived caring for others, helping one another, and receiving aid from the world as very meaningful; they talked about a modification of attitudes and found meaning through an acceptance of blind fate; they were convinced that they were even stronger for having survived the quake, which is consistent with research findings addressing the coping patterns of the Armenian survivors of the Ottoman Turkish Genocide (Kalayjian, Gergerian, Shahinian, & Saraydarian, 1995). They were convinced that they were indomitable, echoing the words of Nietzsche: "That which does not kill me makes me stronger."

Survivors who found meaning in their trauma measured much lower on the Reaction Index Scale. They also reached acceptance, which is essential in the move toward resolving an existential crisis. The acceptance stage, as defined by Kubler-Ross (1969), is neither happy nor sad. It is devoid of feeling; a passive acquiescence to the tragic triad of human existence: pain, guilt, and death (Frankl, 1962).

Commitment and Faith in the Earth.   As respondents with meaninglessness focused on the past and asked, "Why us? What have we done to deserve this?", implying that trauma and disaster happen to bad people, the ones with meaning focused on the present moment and the meaningful experiences they gained by helping and receiving help from one another. They expressed hope for the future, stating, "Look at how the world has come to help us (the

Armenians); the closed Soviet system has opened its doors; there is more communication, caring, and connectedness." These survivors expressed a moral and emotional commitment as well as a faith toward their environment and Mother Earth. They expressed commitment to restore and to rebuild, not only to bring their environment to the predisaster state, but to make it even "better" and "safer." According to Goldsmith (1993), a moral and emotional commitment is required to preserve the critical order of the Earth or the biosphere, as well as faith in our capacity to develop cultural patterns that will enable us to maintain the integrity and stability of the natural world.

THERAPEUTIC INTERVENTIONS

Therapeutic interventions utilized included art therapy, biofeedback, bibliotherapy, the coloring storybook, drawings (structured and unstructured), family therapy, group therapy, instruction booklets, logotherapy, mediation, play therapy, pharmacotherapy, and short-term psychodynamic psychotherapy. No single clinical intervention would have been successful to treat all post-quake symptomatology.

When I asked survivors what helped them cope with the impact of the earthquake and what they considered as caring behaviors, surprisingly—or perhaps not surprisingly—they mentioned first and foremost "being there," "caring," and "listening." The majority of the survivors identified listening as a very helpful caring behavior. This is consistent with my research findings on spouses of cancer patients (Kalayjian, 1989). Listening is recognized as a major therapeutic attitude in effective communication process (Ruesch, 1975). Other caring behaviors identified were: talking, touching, holding hands, and allowing expression of feelings.

The second most frequently mentioned caring behavior was providing information on subjects of primary concern: governmental involvement; basic needs such as shelter, food, and clothing; the possibilities for future plans. This response was consistent with the responses of Hurricane Andrew survivors in Southern Florida, as well as earthquake survivors in Southern California.

CONCLUSION

Disaster impact reduction is an immense task that no one country, or no one organization can achieve alone. It requires an ongoing commitment for communication, cooperation, and collaboration. It requires responsibility to change—not a first-order change, where there is only a superficial attempt to modify things, but a second-order change, where there is a deeper organizational change (Watzlawick, Beavin, & Jackson, 1967).

Responsibility implies a sense of obligation to oneself, to the Earth, and to others around us. We as nurses and caregivers are in key positions to empower our clients by helping them uncover, discover, or recover their responsibility. We can empower them and help them become free but yet connected to their emotions, environment, and soul; free from moral conflicts and a conflict of conscience, which—according to Frankl (1986)—can lead to an existential neurosis. We can help ourselves and others to find this freedom through logotherapy—finding meaning—in the situations that we encounter.

Pain and suffering caused by natural or human-induced disasters may cause a fruitful tension, making us aware of what ought not be (Frankl, 1986); helping us to come together and act responsibly and collectively; making us not only understand our obligations to one another and to the Earth, but also to *feel* such obligations; and above all, making us care and exhibit our caring in a therapeutic way.

Let us integrate our soma, psyche, and spirit. Let's harmonize our thinking, feeling, and meaning. If these three functions are torn apart, thinking deteriorates into schizoid intellectual activity, via technological haphazard advancements; feeling deteriorates into neurotic life-damaging passions, exhibited by depression and suicide (Fromm, 1993); and meaning is replaced with an existential void or spiritual emptiness (Frankl, 1986).

PERSONAL STATEMENT

I believe in the importance of respecting and caring for our environment as we care and respect ourselves and fellow human beings.

As a graduate student at Columbia University, I pursued my interest in environmental issues. I read extensively on the Gaian principle. I firmly believe that if we poison our environment we poison ourselves. Thus, it is very clear that if hospitals discard syringes and other medical waste hastily, it will soon appear on our shores; or if we seed the soil with mines and unexploded bomb shells (as in Vietnam), even a quarter century later, unwary farmers would be killed or severely injured.

In my capacity as co-founder of the Mental Health Outreach Program for Armenia, having traveled thrice to Armenia after the devastating earthquake of 1988, I was touched by the profound reverence with which Armenians related to their ancestral land. I witnessed many a citizen kneeling humbly and kissing the ground (the soil), as though every square inch of it were holy.

This deep, powerful, and spiritual link between a human being and the earth underscores the indispensability of the health of the planet to the health of humanity.

REFERENCES

Adler, A. (1980). *What life should mean to you.* London: Oxford University Press. Original work published in 1932.

Alfaro, R. (1986). *Application of nursing process: A step-by-step guide.* Philadelphia: Lippincott.

Allaby, M. (1989). *A guide to Gaia.* New York: Dutton.

American Psychiatric Association. (1994). *Diagnostic and statistical manual of mental disorders* (4th ed.). Washington, DC: Author.

Bolin, R. (1989). Natural disasters. In R. Giest & B. Lubin (Eds.), *Psychosocial aspects of disaster* (pp. 61–85). New York: Wiley.

Christou, E. (1976). *The logos of the soul.* Zurich, Switzerland: Springer Publications.

Fabry, J. (1980). *The pursuit of meaning.* San Francisco: Harper & Row.

Frankl, V. E. (1969). *The will to meaning.* New York: New American Library.

Frankl, V. E. (1978). *The unheard cry for meaning.* New York: Simon & Schuster.

Frankl, V. E. (1984). *Man's search for meaning.* New York: Simon & Schuster.

Frankl, V. E. (1986). *The doctor and the soul.* New York: Vintage Books.

Frederick, C. J. (1986). *Children traumatized by catastrophic situation.* In S. Eth & R. Pynoos (Eds.), *Posttraumatic stress disorder in children.* Washington, DC: American Psychiatric Press.

Fromm, E. (1969). *Escape from freedom.* New York: Avon Books.

Goldsmith, E. (1963). *The way: An ecological world-view.* Boston: Shambhala.

IE/PAC (1992). *Hazard identification and evaluation in a local community.* Technical Report Series No. 12, United Nations Environmental Program. Paris: Industry & Environment Program Activity Center.

Jung, C. (1972). Vom werden der personlichkeit. In D. Leontiev, The meaning crisis in Russia today. *The International Forum for Logotherapy, 15*(1), 41–45.

Kalayjian, A. S., Gergerian, E., Shahinian, S., & Saraydarian, L. (1995). Coping with genocide: An exploration of the experience of Armenian survivors. *Journal for Traumatic Stress.*

Kalayjian, A. S. (1994a, November/December). A mental health outreach program following the earthquake in Armenia: Utilizing the nursing process in developing and managing a post-natural-disaster plan. *Issues in Mental Health Nursing, 15*(6).

Kalayjian, A. S. (1994b). *Disaster management manual.* Longbranch, NJ: Vista Publishing, Inc.

Kalayjian, A. S. (1991, October). *Genocide, earthquake, and ethnic turmoil: Multiple traumas of a nation.* Paper presented at the 7th Annual Convention of the International Society for Traumatic Stress Studies, Washington, DC.

Kalayjian, A. S. (1989). Coping with cancer. The spouse's perspective. *Archives of Psychiatric Nursing, III*(3), 166–172.

Leontiev, D. (1992). The meaning crisis in Russia today. *The International Forum for Logotherapy, 15*(1), 41–45.

Levinson, J. (1989). Existential vacuum in grieving widows. *International Forum for Logotherapy 12*(2), 48–51.

Lovelock, J. E. (1979). *Gaia: A new look at life on earth.* Oxford, England: Oxford University Press.

Quarantelli, E. L. (1985). Social support systems: Some behavioral patterns in the context of mass evacuation action. In B. Sowdor (Ed.), *Disasters and mental health: Selected contemporary perspectives* (DHHS Publication No. ADM 85-1421, 122-136). Washington, DC: U.S. Government Printing Office.

Reusch, J. (1975). *Therapeutic Communication.* New York: Norton.

Sorensen, J., et al. (1987). *The impacts of hazardous technology: The psychosocial effects of restarting TMI-I.* New York: SUNY Press.

Sullivan, W. (1988, December). Pressing rock masses mark center of quake. *New York Times.*

United Nations Environment Program. (1993–1994). *Environment data report.* Oxford, England: Blackwell Publishers.

Valdov, E. (1993). *Peace and the environment: Saving humanity and our home—the Earth.* Paper presented at Awards Day, Pace University School of Nursing, Pleasantville, New York.

von Bertalanffy, L. (1970) Chance or law. In A. Koestler & J. R. Smythies (Eds.), *Beyond reductionism* (p. 149). New York: Macmillan.

Watzlawick, P., Beavin, J. H., & Jackson, D. D. (1967). *Pragmatics of human communication: A study of interactional patterns, pathologies, and paradoxes.* New York: Norton.

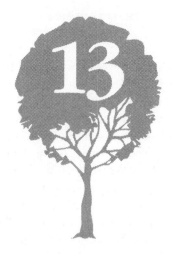

Environments Experienced by Hospital Nurses during Hurricane Andrew

Marcia Dombro

I n 1992, the focus of the Nursing Education Department at Baptist Hospital of Miami was to provide an educational environment that promoted excellent nursing practice. During and immediately after Hurricane Andrew, on August 24, 1992, this focus was urgently expanded to include concern for caring environments for nurses as they were continuing to care for patients under environmental conditions rarely imagined in our nation. This chapter presents descriptions of hospital and personal living environments of nurses, and actions taken to create and support caring environments for living and working in nursing during this disaster. The author was the Director of Nursing Education at Baptist Hospital during the time period described. Reflections, illustrations, recommendations, and questions for research are included.

Are nurses consciously aware of the hospital environment where they work? This may seem, at first, a foolish question, but there is much in our work lives that we notice only when there is a problem. For example, a damaged hospital painfully makes visible the usually transparent everyday functions that must be performed to maintain a health-promoting and caring environment.

Nurse philosophers and theorists of the 1990s talk about caring as the essence of nursing (Watson, 1988, p. 33). Caring is not a totally internal and subjective type of experience; it is characterized by interactivity with the environment where it takes place. Sympathy and empathy can occur within an individual without any knowledge of or effect on the subjects of these feelings. Caring, in the context of nursing, however, implies that some action or response has taken place, which can lead the patient in a positive direction. A great deal of caring was, and still is, needed in Miami because of Hurricane Andrew.

LIVING AND WORKING BEFORE THE HURRICANE

Baptist Hospital is a 513-bed, not-for-profit institution located in unincorporated Dade County. This area, called Kendall, is south of the city of Miami and serves mostly middle- to upper-middle-income people. Many hospital employees had purchased homes here. Others lived further south, in Homestead or the Redlands, areas that are more rural than suburban.

The meaning environment at Baptist Hospital encouraged and rewarded quality in every area. Employees were proud of working there, and the corporate culture of excellence was nurtured in every possible way. The environment was luxurious, and supplies were plentiful. There was great loyalty to the institution and to excellent patient care. "The world view of a culture can be defined as that which provides the basic assumptions and the total attitude of life. It is the meaning environment that envelops individuals; it presents the conceptual and interpretive organizing patterns that individuals integrate into their own meaning-creating process" (Polkinghorn, 1983, p. 28).

PREPARING FOR THE HURRICANE

One predictable thing about hurricanes is that there are several days' warning, and preparations for a safe environment can be made. Weather mapping showed that the hospital was located directly in the path of the storm. Once this was determined, hospital administration immediately went into action to make arrangements for what was to come. A supply of water was prepared. Debris was cleared from building projects that were in progress. Anything that might blow away was taken down or secured. Trees were pruned of branches that might break off and become projectiles. Sandbags were placed around doors and windows where water could seep in. Large areas of glass were protected with boards or plywood.

Preparation of the staff began as soon as it was certain that the hospital would be directly affected.

[The first department head and managers' meeting was on Sunday, August 23] at 11 A.M., shortly after the hurricane was upgraded to a level 5 status. . . . Among the expectations: The hospital w[ould] have enough fuel on hand to provide generator power for approximately four days. Water pressure w[ould] be lost. No one w[ould] be able to flush toilets or obtain tap water. Internal phone extensions and paging systems . . . [would] remain operational, but service for incoming and outgoing calls . . . [might] be lost. . . . [W]hether or not they are ill, [hundreds of] people [would come to the hospital] seeking shelter. At the meeting, [each area was asked] to have two teams of staffing in the hospital by midnight—one team to work, one to sleep. . . . That goal was vital: to bring in staff . . . in advance of the storm, since they might have trouble getting [t]here afterwards. . . .

Everyone made their phone calls, then went home to prepare their homes as best they could. . . . [They said goodbye to their families and then returned] to work. It was a very hard thing to do.

The Hurricane Command Post in Nursing Administration—staffed by vice presidents on a rotational schedule—

. . . [was] activated. [Two hundred pregnant women showed]
up for shelter. . . . Food Services prepare[d] thousands of
sandwiches. . . . Purchasing and Warehouse staff move[d]
vital supplies into the hospital. . . . [T]he first of many hur-
ricane bulletins [was delivered] to employees. As midnight
approache[d] and preparations continue[d], people tr[ied]
to grab a few hours sleep—on office floors, on lounge
chairs. (Sylver, 1992, p. 2)

LIVING AND WORKING AFTER THE HURRICANE

At least three-fourths of the 3,500 employees at Baptist Hospital
had homes that were significantly damaged or were rendered totally uninhabitable. Many had sought refuge in closets or bath-
rooms while they listened to their homes being ripped apart. What
they had left was a tangle of broken debris, glass, and possessions.

Baptist Hospital was the closest fully functioning hospital to the
disaster area. The workload was tremendous until volunteer help
came. This is how the emergency room was described on the
morning after the hurricane:

By 9:30 A.M. the Emergency Center is wall-to-wall people.
Computers are down. There is no water, no air condition-
ing. It is so hot and humid, the floors are sweating. . . . "There
were so many injured people. Lots of lacerations, broken
bones and wounds related to people going through the
wreckage of their homes. Coronaries due to the incredible
stress." . . . As the hours fly past, all awareness of title has dis-
appeared, [n]urses from . . . all hospital departments work
next to administrators, physicians, patients, and relatives,
helped by volunteers and secretaries. (Sylver, 1992, p. 2)

By Friday, the emergency room had seen about 2,500 people,
which amounted to 500 patients per day.

The overall hospital census, which was usually around 385, was
not much lower after the storm. This was an important issue because of potentially limited supplies and services. It was difficult

to move patients out because many of them had no homes to return to. Some devastated nursing homes had no choice but to bring their patients into the hospital. When the volume of patients began to rise, some were sent to other hospitals further to the north.

Two weeks after the hurricane, a nurse described her working conditions this way:

> *It was a very, very difficult situation. Feelings are still flying all around the rooms, I mean emotions are very high. I had a doctor cry in my arms the other day who I didn't even know. . . . He lost his home [and] something had happened to his wife, an accident from the hurricane . . . she was injured . . . Basically, we're suppressing what's happened to us so we can care for others . . . and then, slowly, I think that . . . emotions are surfacing . . . at awkward times. . . . I didn't even know this doctor, and he just . . . burst out crying. I really don't know how to sum it up, it's still so much a part of everybody's life and I think that it's going to be for at least another year or so.*

MAKING CONNECTIONS AFTER THE HURRICANE

Communication became the crucial web connecting people and securing the environment. Immediately after the storm, at least 75% of the phones were out of order, so that nurses who were working could not call home. People were urged to call local radio stations for assistance if they had not heard from family members. Many internal communication tools were used in the hospital such as: *Vocal Chord, Employee Assistance Memos, NurseGram, Friday Update.*

Connecting People with One Another

Administration with Employees.   There was a concerted effort to make sure that hospital communication flowed freely in all directions. Devastating changes had occurred in the personal life of nearly every employee. To keep the hospital functioning, there was no way to ignore the interaction between private and professional worlds. People had to be allowed the flexibility to begin putting their lives back together. This was acknowledged and supported at every level of the organization.

Department Heads/Managers with Employees. Department heads and managers were seen as linking the outside world, the hospital as an institution, and individual employees. Employees viewed department heads and managers as sources of strength and information, and assumed that they were able to cope: they needed to be urged to take time out for personal and family needs, because most of them slept in the hospital and worked for extended periods without a break.

Daily meetings informed managers about which services/departments had changed and what functions were still available. There were frequent updates on the latest news, because the status of the rest of the community affected the hospital. Many managers were too busy to watch television or listen to the radio. Their personal information about the disaster often came from patients. One manager said that she was not fully aware of the devastation outside until Wednesday, when she was finally able to leave for a short time, to look at her house.

The normal functioning of the community was monitored as it began to move again. Hours of operation of open businesses were shared. For example, no pharmacies were open after 5 P.M., and only certain gas stations and supermarkets were open.

The hospital had been scheduled for a hospital accreditation visit during the next few months. Managers were very worried about this. Administration contacted the accrediting agency and arranged for the visit to be rescheduled.

Employees with One Another. Many nurses were very concerned when their colleagues did not reappear within a few days after the storm. Each nursing unit had its own system of networking, to find out what had happened to employees. There was particular concern for the large numbers of people who lived in the Homestead area, where the damage was known to be particularly devastating. The grapevine was humming with news of people who had been unaccounted for. Some units even enlisted the police to check on the welfare of those who could not otherwise be found.

Staffing Office with Nurses.   Staffing was a tremendous problem in the first few days after the hurricane. I made 33 calls for the emergency room, but was able to contact only three people who could work and were not trapped in their homes by downed trees and debris. For the first week or so, the staffing office was simply trying to find people. A staffing inventory was an ongoing task for several weeks.

Three days after the hurricane, volunteer nurses began arriving by bus and were met by a cheering but exhausted crowd. They poured in from Tampa, West Palm Beach, and Jacksonville, and from other states. Many of these nurses slept on mattresses on the floors in the hospital auditorium and classrooms. Because of the large number of volunteers, the governor of Florida gave a special waiver on nursing and medical licenses, to allow volunteers to work if they were credentialed in another state.

By September 8, two weeks after the storm, the hospital was back to 90% of normal staffing levels, but there was great anxiety about what would happen when the volunteers went home. By September 14th, 82% of employees had returned and 18% had resigned; however, many of those who were working could not be there full-time. They needed to be able to periodically leave work to make repairs on their houses and to deal with contractors.

Families with One Another.   Without electricity and phone service, the only widely available mass communication system left consisted of battery-powered radios and televisions, which broadcast information about families searching for one another. The author met a woman who had been pulled from her demolished home by Emergency Medical Technicians. She had nothing but the clothing she was wearing. The only family she had was a sister in New Jersey. She could not remember their telephone number, and she was so upset that she had trouble remembering their last name. Many long-distance phone calls were needed to make the connection. The same scenario was played out many times during the early days after the hurricane.

Nursing Students with Instructors. Nursing students called the Nursing Education office to obtain information about their instructors, because nursing schools were closed. Nursing instructors also called for information about students and staff.

Patients with Their Physicians. Locating physicians—and all of the other health care workers at the hospital—was a major problem. Physicians had the same proportion of damage to their homes as everyone else, but many of them also suffered destruction to their offices. Temporary office space was made available for many of them in the hospital or the adjacent office building. Patients called the hospital, unable to think of any other way to find their doctors. One nurse had the specific task of walking through the hospital halls to locate physicians and record their telephone numbers and temporary addresses.

Connecting People with Resources

Every kind of community resource was needed by employees. Healing the nursing environment included healing the nurse. People needed to know the most basic information: what stores and gas stations were open or closed, and how to contact community agencies. Any kind of travel was at first hazardous and sometimes impossible because of flooding, downed power lines, and trees. No one could drive around aimlessly looking for something that was open. Some people, in fact, were trapped in their homes with no access to outside assistance for several days. Employees were allowed to use hospital phones to make essential personal calls. Telephone numbers were distributed for services such as Fire Rescue, Health Hotline, Environmental Hotline, and Suicide Hotline. Insurance company numbers were also distributed, because address books and other papers had been lost in the storm.

Connecting People with Volunteer Help. Nursing units were so overwhelmed that it was difficult for them to think creatively about how they could use untrained people. A volunteer desk was set up, and a representative who knew the capabilities of the volunteers toured the units to make suggestions about how they could be of help.

Sometimes, patients themselves volunteered to help.

*Monday afternoon a fire [broke] out in the elevator shaft
near Pediatrics. [The] . . . Pediatric Nurse Manager [said]:
"Teenage patients were carrying babies, helping us get them
out. The whole floor had to get over to the Tower [Building].
It was so hot. I kept thinking: 'This is all we need.' But everyone was great, and after an hour, we were able to go back so
things could return to normal—well, make that 'hurricane-
normal.' The kids had already been frightened. Rain, wind
and fire. We had it all. But the children were safe."* (Vocal
Chord, *1993, p. 5)*

POSTHURRICANE CARE OF
THE WORKING ENVIRONMENT

Creating and supporting caring environments began with concern
for safe, dry, and clean surroundings, which seemed at the same
time both simple and luxurious.

Safety

Because the hospital was built to withstand hurricanes, it was one
of the safest structures in the area. Glass doors and windows were
of special concern because they could have been (and were) damaged by flying debris and roof tiles. Broken glass was rapidly
cleared away, and windows were repaired. Trees and debris outside were cleared away with the help of the National Guard. Because of the lack of air conditioning in the hospital, the
environment was no longer safe for cardiac patients from the critical care unit, so they were transferred to other hospitals.

Dryness

People lived with crumbling walls, leaking roofs, no air conditioning, no electricity, and no water, yet they still came in to work.
Things were so upset at home that they felt it was a relief to come
to the hospital, where at least it was dry. An environmental services

workers said: "I didn't have insurance, and I lost my house in Cutler Ridge and everything in it. Thanks to the Sunshine Fund, I've gotten money to replace all my windows. So at least I'm dry now. And I've gotten the roof back on my home" (*Vocal Chord,* 1993, p. 3).

Cleanliness/Infection Control

Clean Environment. Because many of the environmental service workers lived in Homestead, where the worst devastation had taken place, there were very few people available for cleaning and trash removal. All available employees had to do this, with the help of volunteers.

Clean Water. After the hurricane, radio and television programs urged citizens to avoid using showers or brushing teeth with water from the tap. Because of the nature of the water table in southern Florida, the heat, and the humidity, there was a danger of contamination of water, which could lead to water-borne epidemics such as typhoid fever and cholera.

The hospital water supply came from City of Miami water mains, and could not be used until the all-clear was given nine days after the hurricane. As nurses, we learn that one of our most basic responsibilities is protection from infection. With tap water banned for both drinking and washing, an alcohol-based product, which did not require water, was used for hand rinsing. Having no water to clean patients and to wash hands is almost unthinkable. According to Heidegger, "We understand human action—and act ourselves—within a background of practices (bodily, personal, and cultural) that is always present, although it can never be made fully explicit" (cited in Packer, 1985, p. 1087). Both patients and nurses take for granted that they will use water to clean themselves every day. One nurse described the problem of patient hygiene: "We had bottled water, [but] you don't want to use a whole bottle of . . . drinking water on a patient, to bathe. So you have to really get back to basics. . . . Peri[neal] care and the more important things take precedence . . . ."

Precautions were taken to avoid using any potentially contaminated water from drinking fountains, ice machines, and dialysis machines. Even toilet flushing was restricted because of low water pressure and limited amounts of water in hospital holding tanks.

Keeping employees healthy required education in safe water use at home, and this information was disseminated in many ways.

Electricity

Nurses were advised to turn off anything possible, to conserve electricity. Worst of all, there was no air conditioning in the 90° heat. Full power was not restored until September 8, fifteen days after the storm.

Miami became a different city after the advent of air conditioning, something that no one notices until it is gone. One nurse, who developed a new appreciation for it after the hurricane, said: "You know, air conditioning was such a luxury, it was unbelievable." Here is a description of what happened to the Surgery Center as a result of damage from the storm and no air conditioning:

> . . . *All day Monday, water pour[ed] through the ceiling. Without air conditioning and full sterilization capabilities, procedures [were] limited to emergencies, and performed in one room only, where the temperature under the lights [was] well above 90 degrees. . . . Sending people in there [was] like punishment. Surgeons and nurses came out of that room without a dry thread of clothing on their bodies. . . . The lights would flicker on and off; [they] had to use backup battery lights and a few fans to help cool things down a little. (Sylver, 1992, p. 5)*

POSTHURRICANE CARE OF EMPLOYEE BASIC NEEDS

"The ideal and value of caring is clearly not just a *thing* out there, but is a starting point, a stance, an attitude, which has to become a will, an intention, a commitment, and a conscious judgment that manifests itself in concrete acts" (Watson, 1988, p. 32). After the hurricane, a hospital commitment had to be made about what resources and time should be allocated to meet the desperate and vastly increased needs of employees. The decision was that everything possible would be done to help meet the basic needs that people were temporarily unable to take care of themselves.

Immediately after the hurricane, shelter for homeless employees was provided adjacent to the hospital, in an empty building undergoing renovation. Any suitable unoccupied hospital floor space was used for sleeping. The usual concepts of homelessness were inadequate for the conditions of nurses and other staff. Some common synonyms for homeless are: vagrant, outcast, itinerant, derelict. None of these is applicable to people who are made homeless by a disaster of this magnitude. The meaning of the word had changed for those who were trying to count the numbers of homeless or to find housing for them. Numbers were very difficult to determine, but it was estimated that as many as 1,500 employees had no fit dwelling place. There were many generous offers from Miamians whose houses were spared, but the homeless did not want to live with people they did not know, even when it was rent-free. Some people moved in with their own extended family members and, although their houses were destroyed, did not consider themselves homeless. Others continued to live on their land until their houses were condemned and they were forced to move.

Sometimes, one room was left untouched when the rest of the house was destroyed. The residents did not consider themselves homeless, even when the open sky may have been the living room "ceiling." Some roofs were blown off without causing water damage inside, because Andrew was a "dry hurricane." However, the torrential rains that followed during the next few days damaged whatever was left. Wet walls and remaining possessions soon began to grow mold and mildew in the humidity and heat. Nevertheless, people hung onto their dwellings, no matter how uncomfortable the situation became. It was as though their identities would be lost if they left the remains of their former lives. "We know ourselves only indirectly through the things we have made, the objectified or fixed residues of our thoughts in physical things like buildings or tools" (Dilthey, 1988, p. 27). Because people were clinging to damaged and dangerous surroundings, speedy repair became more pressing than it would have been had home owners elected to move out.

There were other reasons for people's decisions to stay under unbearable conditions. Supervision of large-scale repairs required constant attention. In some areas, there was a problem with looters, especially at night. People who had rifles slept with them by their beds. Some families had lost animals and were trying to find them, or they were afraid that apartment houses would not allow pets. Many had followed their pets to safety during the hurricane.

FEMA (Federal Emergency Management Agency) came to the hospital to provide allowances for temporary housing, but any housing was difficult to find. Trailers were available, but presented a logistic and zoning problem. Almost nothing was available in Dade County after nearly 150,000 homes had been destroyed. A nurse from Baptist's neuro-orthopedic floor said, "Out of our staff, one-third lost their homes. It was quite amazing to see that, after that, they could come in and provide such quality care to the . . . casualties of the hurricane."

Assistance was given in many tangible ways, including home repair, a food bank, a clothing bank, child care, and transportation to and from the hospital. Financial assistance was also given in the form of immediate cash advances, special loans, and unusual handling of benefit time.

EXPRESSIONS OF CARING IN
THE DISASTER ENVIRONMENT

Working environments included compassion in each word, touch, and step—concern for other was the context of each action. Caring overrode the continuous uncertainty inherent in the post-hurricane environment. "Human caring in nursing, . . . is not just an emotion, or concern, attitude or benevolent desire. Caring is the moral ideal of nursing whereby the end is protection, enhancement, and preservation of human dignity" (Watson, 1988, p. 29). The indignities suffered by victims of the hurricane included a loss of control over their own life spaces, an important contributor to negative feelings experienced in a crisis. "[Crisis] involves a sense of being overwhelmed and a weakening in the individual's ability to act autonomously and effectively. A sense of identity diffusion (the individual's lack of a sense of who he is and where he is going) is often experienced . . ." (Barten, 1971, p. 30). For many employees, the only "normal" place left in their lives was the workplace, where they could continue to function nearly as they had before. The caring they found at work helped to sustain them when they returned to the devastation awaiting them at home.

Expressions of confidence and caring from administration gave employees some of the autonomy they had lost in their personal lives. The Vice President for Nursing sent an inspiring letter to every nursing employee in the hospital. She continually made her presence known by daily visits to nursing units and frequent expressions of her concern for each individual. "When the staff observe[s] the nursing leadership taking a calm and controlled approach, they [are] reassured and able to generalize this sense of order and safety to the patients" (Nordberg, 1993, p. 25).

Business was definitely altered by administration to more appropriately fit the situation. Instead of an annual awards banquet, employees were allowed to spend the money on items from a catalog. The annual Christmas basket contest was also changed. Hospital work units produced fifty-two beautifully decorated baskets with gifts and food for entire families. These were usually donated to the poor, but this year, they were given to employees.

Each department head was asked to keep a log of significant events, including a list of people who had gone above and beyond the call of duty. Many of the department heads themselves should have been on the list.

Nurse managers also submitted to the department heads a list of people who had done outstanding things. Each nurse manager made sure that work schedules were flexible so that people could take care of personal needs. One nurse described the role of her manager in this way: "On this floor, we have a great nurse manager who also had considerable damage and has a very good heart . . . and she's really taken time to try to be individually with each nurse, and try to do the best she can, or whatever she can for the nurses who have really suffered."

Peers would support one another in countless ways. One of these ways was the use of humor. Humor is a very effective way to relieve stress and to put unpleasant situations into perspective. This was officially part of the corporate culture, to the extent that a humor committee was responsible for encouraging laughter at every level of the organization. Many volunteer nurses made note of the ability of nurses to maintain a sense of humor in the midst of the disaster. Nurse Network, the professional newsletter, contained cartoons that were based on some real happenings.

Gratitude to volunteer health care workers was strongly felt by nurses. The hospital Recruitment and Retention Committee addressed this feeling about four months after the storm. There had been a total of about 400 volunteers—nurses, respiratory therapists, and physical therapists came from all over the country. A thank-you package, sent to each of them, contained items with the

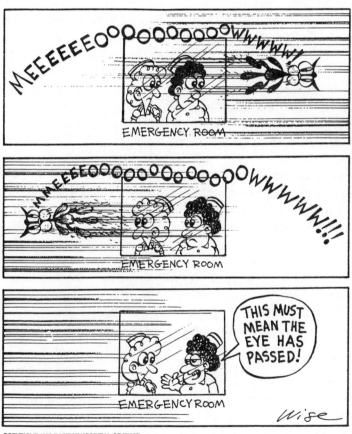

Baptist Hospital logo: lunch boxes, watches, umbrellas, along with mementoes and brochures from the hospital.

Many letters received by the hospital expressed the caring of the volunteer nurses and the personal satisfaction they found in being able to be of assistance during the disaster.

Health care workers showed their true commitment to patients during this time. Prior to the hurricane, the hospital corporate culture conveyed a sense of "hospitality" and caring to everyone who entered. Even under the difficult conditions surrounding the hurricane, this ethos remained strong. All areas were affected—perhaps most dramatically, the emergency room:

> *The patients just kept coming. . . . It was unbelievable. But our staff, . . . couldn't bring themselves to leave. Some worked 36 hours straight; others, even longer. The outpouring of compassion they showed to these patients, despite the losses they'd suffered themselves. . . . They'd try to find out where someone else's relatives might be, without knowing where their own relatives were. They'd listen to horror stories, come into the office to cry and hug each other, then go back out again. (Sylver, 1992, p. 2)*

There were many extraordinary services provided for patients. For example, after being admitted to the floors, those who were especially frightened were given individualized attention; volunteers were asked to just sit and talk with them so that they would not be alone.

Stress Management

Posthurricane Debriefing.   It was immediately evident that each of the 3,500 employees in the hospital would be subjected to tremendous stress as a result of the disaster. Because they were part of the devastated community, all of them were victims; but as health care workers, they were simultaneously expected to act as rescuers. They spent their workdays taking care of others, and then had to go home to put back together their own shattered lives. An approach was needed that would reach as many employees as possible and create a general atmosphere of caring, understanding, and support for one another during the difficult days ahead.

The concept of a "Critical Incident Stress Debriefing Team," developed by the U.S. Public Health Service and the University of Maryland, seemed to be the answer. It was hoped that this would reduce the incidence of posttraumatic stress disorder. Stress debriefing allows people to reveal themselves and their true experiences during the hurricane to their coworkers in a nonjudgmental and supportive atmosphere. The debriefer is a model for helpful communication with others, and teaches the work group how to recognize and support others when signs of posthurricane stress appear. Managers who had read a handbook prepared by the Human Resources Department, *Normal People Having Normal Reactions to an Abnormal Situation,* supported debriefing. The handbook helped them to recognize signs of stress in their staff and in themselves, and to see how outside assistance might make a difference.

The creation of the debriefing team involved selecting individuals with counseling skills, either from inside the institution or from among the outside volunteers, to lead hurricane discussion groups on every shift, on every unit in the hospital. This group included nursing education staff, volunteer social workers, psychologists, and others. They were given special training to conduct these sessions.

The debriefers found that it was a tremendously draining experience to enter the lives of 12 to 15 staff members at a time and to share the details of their suffering. All debriefers took a supply of tissues with them because, invariably, the tears would come when coworkers heard heart-rending stories for the first time. No matter how devastating their situation, nurses would nearly always add the postscript, "Other people had it much worse than we did." The debriefing teams had one session together, where, with the help of psychologists and social workers, they discussed their own feelings. More than 1,100 employees participated during 118 debriefing sessions.

Counseling.   Administration expected that reactions to the stress of the hurricane and the postdisaster life disruptions would include

an increase in all types of stress-related problems, including substance abuse and family violence. Counseling was made available in
the hospital, on a voluntary basis, by a cadre of psychologists, social workers, and family therapists. There was no charge, so that
anyone who needed these individualized services would feel free to
use them. Managers were encouraged to recommend counseling to
employees whom they identified as having difficulty coping.

After the initial period of shock and numbness wore off, the
ever-present reality of hurricane-related stress became evident.
Most outside help had dwindled after hospital functioning began
to return to something near normal. The personal lives of most
employees, however, were far from normal. One employee spoke
about her feelings: "We're surviving. My experience has probably
caused me to look at my life a little closer and realize the importance of relationships. We are changing our priorities to concen-
trate more on family things rather than material things" (Sylver,
1993, p. 4). A special half-day program was given on October 9,
1992, to help employees deal with their relationships with children and other family members.

Five months after the storm, Baptist Hospital was a corporate
sponsor for a series of talks called "Strong in the Broken Places."
The speaker was Landon Saunders. He began by asking people to
share some of the feelings that the hurricane had prompted in
them. Some responses were: anxiety, anger, frustration, terror,
helplessness, upheaval, sadness, disorientation, grief, loss, guilt,
being overwhelmed, dislocation, happiness. The last reaction
came from someone who said that he was happy simply to have
survived the disaster.

Saunders pointed out that it is not so much what actually happens that determines the effect on us; it is how we see what happens. Our view of the world determines our experience in it. "What
is essential in human existence is that the human has transcended
nature—yet remains a part of it. The human can go forward through
the use of the mind to higher levels of consciousness by finding
meaning and harmony in existence" (Watson, 1988, p. 45).

One remnant of the hurricane employees would wish to keep:
the sense of camaraderie and mutual support that they felt. When
I asked one nurse what helped her the most to keep going during

the hurricane, she said: "I think . . . it was that everybody seemed to realize that we were all in it together, and human nature and kindness took over. And I hope it doesn't leave."

Health care workers are constantly battling the destructive potential of disease. Drugs and treatments give the illusion that primal nature can be bounded, reined in, and conquered. Those who experienced the overwhelming power of Hurricane Andrew were humbled by its force and had to recognize the importance of their understanding of and cooperation with nature. They have also been forever changed in relation to their attitudes about the relative unimportance of material things and the primacy of creating and nurturing caring human connections with one another.

PERSONAL STATEMENT

People, like myself, who live in Miami, Florida, know that there is an intensity about the weather here that can catch the unwary. Sudden drenching rainstorms obscure vision and stop traffic. Small tornadoes have touched down to ravage patio screens on our block. Our street was once so flooded that children paddled by in small boats, using buckets to scoop up disoriented fish from the canal nearby. A vacation on Sanibel Island was once spoiled when the beaches were covered with thousands of dead fish, killed by the "Red Tide." All of this reminds me of our connection with the environment. I know this is a worldwide link when I see a beautiful sunset, aglow with stunning reds, pinks, and oranges. The colors are often influenced by atmospheric dust blown over the ocean from the Sahara Desert. It is impossible to ignore the physical environment in South Florida.

The psychological environment in the workplace became a compelling interest of mine while I was the Director of Nursing Education at Baptist Hospital of Miami. I became convinced that education in the hospital setting involves much more than presenting classes. The working environment influences whether nursing knowledge is used at the bedside or left in class notes. Nurturing this environment as a living thing is an important task of nursing staff developers. Attention must constantly be paid to many aspects of keeping positive and caring feelings alive. For example, a nurse's ability to maintain a caring presence for patients may be impaired by burnout. A new employee's perceptions of the workplace as a caring environment may be permanently colored by experiences during orientation. A student nurse learns something about caring from what graduate nurses do and say. Support for the growth of self and coworkers must be present at all levels in the institution. Just as the body and the mind must be cared for, the physical and psychological environments in a hospital must be constantly attended to, in order for it to foster productivity. There is no time when the nursing environment is more severely tested than during and after a disaster.

REFERENCES

Barten, H. (1971). *Brief therapies.* New York: Behavioral Publications.

Dilthey, W. (1988). *Introduction to the human sciences.* Detroit: Wayne State University Press.

Nordberg, M. (1993, January). Trouble in paradise. *Emergency Medical Services,* 38–39.

Packer, M. (1985, October). Hermeneutic inquiry in the study of human conduct. *American Psychologist,* 1081–1093.

Polkinghorn, D. (1983). *Methodology for the human sciences.* Albany: SUNY Press.

Saunders, L. (1993, February). *Strong in the broken places.* Presentation at Baptist Hospital, Miami, Florida.

Sylver, A. (Ed.). (1992, October). *Vocal Chord.* Baptist Hospital of Miami.

Sylver, A. (Ed.). (1993, January). *Vocal Chord.* Baptist Hospital of Miami.

Watson, J. (1988). *Nursing: Human science and human care, a theory of nursing.* New York: National League for Nursing.

Voluntary Simplicity: Nurses Creating a Healing Environment

Kathleen Musker

INTRODUCTION

A s nurses, our primary concern is health. The models of health that we utilize in our work will affect the kind of care we give. In this chapter, I suggest that, from a holistic, systems point of view, the way we care for ourselves and our personal environment will affect the way we care for others and our larger environment. The model I propose is called Voluntary Simplicity, and it was described by Duane Elgin in 1981. It advocates a holistic, ecological life-style, providing an integrated framework for living that incorporates awareness of inner and outer environments. It also provides physical and nonphysical guidelines to help us reconnect with the basic quality of our lives and work.

COMPLEXITY

The complexity of life is no longer a matter of speculation; it is a given. With each passing decade, we become more affected by the complexities of life in our daily lives and jobs. In a culture where more is better, we run faster and faster to keep up with the changes, but somehow the complexities seem to outrun us. In the nonphysical realms, we have religion, mythology, and philosophy to help us understand and cope with life's complexities. In the physical realm, we have science and technology to assist us. Each provides models, maps, and paths to guide us through, but these may become outdated. When this happens, we feel overwhelmed and lost—in need of new models appropriate to our experience and knowledge.

Currently, the mechanistic model of the world is being challenged by the holistic model. The holistic model sees life from a systems perspective in which each system affects the other and is interdependent. We are reexamining our physical and nonphysical models of the world, letting go of those that no longer serve us and identifying new models that are in accord with recent discoveries and our current life-styles.

Holistic theorists now view systems as complex. We live in a world of open, complex systems. We, as human beings, are open, complex systems. The science of complexity attempts to study these systems and theorizes that, out of the apparent chaos of complex systems, a self-organization emerges from contact with both internal and external environments (Davidson & Ray, 1991). Of course, the condition of these environments effects our ability to achieve higher levels of functioning.

Although the study of complex systems is crucial, it is also of value to recognize our ongoing experiential responses to life's complexities. The way in which we respond—for example, with flexibility or rigidity—can make the difference in whether systems develop a pattern of chronic deterioration, or reorganization at a higher level of functioning. The system referred to can be our own personal system, that of our client, or that of the environment.

Nursing theorists Davidson and Ray have applied the science of complexity to nursing research. They suggest that "caring provides the energy by which order evolves out of disorder. In the caring relationship, the goal is to enable the client to evolve his or her own well-being" (1991, p. 83). I would also suggest that it is equally important for the nurse to care for herself and her environment with the same goal in mind.

Watson (1988) considers the human caring process to have an energy field of its own. "It is part of a human consciousness process that can arise from itself, yet it goes beyond itself and becomes part of the life history of each person, as well as part of some larger, deeper, complex pattern of life" (p. 177).

One general response to complexity is "more-is-better." As our currently dominant cultural response, this promotes unchecked growth, a short-term linear view of the consequences of actions. There is a steadily increasing pressure on all life forms, and a sense of urgency. This view relies on "unconsciousness" in various forms. It only seems to work if we ignore some of the unpleasant consequences of our current life-styles such as planetary pollution, poverty, and related illnesses. Personally, we are encouraged to override internal feedback mechanisms, such as physical tension and pain, feelings of anxiety and frustration, and worrisome thoughts that tell us something is wrong. Coping mechanisms generally take the form of suppression of signs and symptoms through one or many addictions. Illness is seen as a problem to get rid of, or, for many, serves as a socially sanctioned way to get off the treadmill. Health care is focused on and primarily values "curing" problems (Burkhardt, 1993). All in all, this is not a response that promotes reorganization of the system at a higher level of functioning.

In the other "less-is-more" response, *quality* is as important as *quantity*. It promotes sustainable growth and a long-term view of the consequences of our actions and decisions. It acknowledges and values all stages of natural cycles, and sees life as a dynamic balance allowing for flexibility, change, and unpredictability. It promotes consciousness through self-reflection, and attends to personal and planetary feedback mechanisms that indicate imbalance. It considers illness and death to be more than unfortunate events:

They're seen as meaningful aspects of health, which, if consciously acknowledged, can lead an individual to reorganization at a higher level of functioning. Health care values both curing and healing. Healing indicates a restoration of the underlying disharmony that characterizes an illness. It values an individual's subjective response to an illness (Burkhardt, 1993).

Each response to complexity can be expressed in many forms, as reflected in cultural norms, institutions, and life-styles. When making a change not yet reflected in mainstream norms, it helps to have maps to guide us. Voluntary simplicity provides this holistic, less-is-more framework.

The holistic principles underlying a shift to voluntary simplicity are from a school of thought that complements nursing theory. They are not something that we have to "add on" to our professional knowledge. They exist within our own profession.

Newman (1986) addresses the paradigm shift to holism in her book *Health as Expanding Consciousness.* From Newman's viewpoint, health is the interaction of the whole person with the environment. The focus of nursing practice is to recognize the pattern of interaction and accept it as a process of evolving consciousness. She views disease as a manifestation of the interactive pattern, not as something separate from it. The objective of nurses within her model is an "authentic involvement of themselves with the patient in a mutual relationship of pattern recognition and augmentation" (Newman, 1986, p. 88). In this model as well as in the caring model of nursing, the person, environment, and health are interconnected, and the totality of each affects the other through simultaneous and continuous interaction (Gaut, 1993). It is not necessary for us to change all the apparently separate parts of our lives in order for a change in the whole to occur.

Watson (1988) wrote, regarding human caring theory, that "transpersonal caring expands the limits of openness and accesses the higher human spirit or field consciousness, therefore it has the capacity to expand human consciousness, transcend the moment, and potentiate healing" (p. 176).

Within the mechanistic model of more-is-better, we typically seek to improve ourselves as nurses by adding on knowledge and skills through seminars, workshops, or advanced degrees. We generally see this knowledge enhancement only as an aspect of our professional lives. Within a holistic model, obtaining more intellectual knowledge is not the only way of enhancing our nursing work; subjective experiences are also of value. The being and doing of our personal lives are inseparable from the being and doing of our professional lives.

Nursing theory and research are validating the holistic paradigm through which integration of the personal and professional are experienced. Rogers's (1970) concept of unitary human beings indicates that human beings and the environment are in continuous, mutual process. Change in one is related to change in the other. Newman (1990) realized that, although caring is an aspect of the nurse–client relationship, it is the *mutuality* of the relationship that is most meaningful. Within this mutuality, both the client and the nurse experience personal transformation or expansion of consciousness. "To be in touch with the other person and the environment, the task is to be in touch with one's own pattern" (Newman, 1986, p. 71).

Self-knowledge, gained through objective, intellectual information as well as through subjective processes, is necessary to learning about one's own pattern. So too is a subtractive mode. Eliminating that which is unnecessary and interferes with our true self-expression or authenticity will enhance our nursing abilities. The attention, self-awareness, and self-nurturing we give our personal lives will directly affect our professional lives. Voluntary simplicity is one way of getting in touch with one's own pattern and, through conscious healthy choices, enhancing well-being for our clients and for our planet.

VOLUNTARY SIMPLICITY

What exactly is voluntary simplicity? It isn't exactly any one thing or one way of living. It is an approach to living that includes greater awareness of what we do, think, and feel in our lives. It involves greater awareness of the consequences of what we do or don't do—consequences for all interconnected, living systems. In

1974, Duane Elgin came upon this description of voluntary simplicity in an article by Richard Gregg, written in 1936:

> *Voluntary simplicity involves both the inner and outer condition. It means singleness of purpose, sincerity and honesty within, as well as avoidance of exterior clutter, of many possessions irrelevant to the chief purpose of life. It means an ordering and guiding of our energy and our desires, a partial restraint in some directions in order to secure greater abundance of life in other directions. It involves a deliberate organization of life for a purpose. (p. 16)*

Voluntary simplicity, as indicated, is both an inner and an outer process. Although there may appear to be less externally as one simplifies, there is more internally as one grows in self-awareness, an inner richness (Elgin, 1981). It balances the "why" of what we do with how we do it.

The internal aspect of voluntary simplicity has to do with "being." It refers to the voluntary component of the process in directing us to reflect on our life's purpose, to become more self-aware (not selfish), to pay attention to what we do, to sort out our wants from our needs, and to hold an intention to act according to personal beliefs and values. It has to do with valuing our inner experience and reconnecting with our authentic selves; we remember who we really are rather than who we appear to be.

The external aspect of voluntary simplicity relates to "doing." It refers to the simplicity component of the process in directing us to act in the world in a life-serving manner. It has to do with acting responsibly—having the ability to respond in a manner congruent with our beliefs, values, and purpose. "Each aspect—living voluntarily and living simply—builds upon the other and promotes the progressive refinement of each. Gradually, the experience of being infuses the process of doing. Life-sensing and life-serving action become one integrated flow of experience. We become whole" (Elgin, 1981, p. 141).

The concept of voluntary simplicity may initially bring to mind images of a spartan life. This and other myths were addressed by Elgin (1981, p. 16).

Myth	Fact
We must live in a rudimentary manner.	Poverty is involuntary. Voluntary simplicity fosters personal empowerment, creativity and a sense of opportunity.
It is a static condition to be achieved.	It is an ever-changing balance, a challenging process.
It means to dogmatically live with less.	It is an intention of living with balance.
It means turning away from progress, a path of no growth.	It is a path of new growth, bringing order, clarity, and purpose.
It requires isolation, living in the country.	It seeks participation and the support of others, making the most of wherever you are.
There is a "right" way to simplify.	It is a relative matter depending on climate, culture, and the character of the individual.

LIVING VOLUNTARILY

The internal aspect of life-style is encompassed by the word *voluntary.* The *American Heritage Dictionary* (1970) defines voluntary as: "acting on one's own initiative. Deliberate, willful action taken with full awareness of the consequences. Any act or work not imposed or demanded by another" (p. 1436).

According to Elgin (1981), "We cannot be intentional when we are not paying attention. We cannot be purposeful when we are not being present. . . . To the extent that we do not notice both inner and outer aspects or our passage through life, then our capacity for voluntary, deliberate, purposeful action will be commensurately diminished" (p. 11).

To act voluntarily has to do with intention—getting off of automatic pilot and into deliberate, thoughtful choices. We are proactive rather than reactive. Clarifying our intention can begin by

asking ourselves simple questions that often have profound answers. In some cases, the responses to early questions lead to a
shifting of intention and new questions. The following beginning
questions were suggested by Elgin (1981, p. 16):

1. Does my work contribute to the well-being of others, or is
   it just a source of income?
2. How much income do I really require?
3. Require for what?
4. How much of my consumption adds to the clutter and complexity of my life rather than to my satisfaction?
5. Are there small changes that I could make in my own life
   that, with may others making similar changes, would result
   in a large difference in the well-being of others?
6. Am I missing much of the richness of life by being preoccupied with the search for social status and consumer
   goods?
7. What is my purpose in life?
8. How am I to take charge of my life?
9. Will my present way of life still be workable when my children grow up?
10. How might their lives, and my own, be different?
11. Am I satisfied with my work?

In order to act in a self-determining manner, we must know ourselves. The truth about our unhealthy habits and imbalances may
not be easy to face, but it is necessary to face them if we are to
reempower ourselves. By our voluntary choice to do this, we can
then assist our clients to reempower themselves, to face and deal
with not only the facts of their illness, but the meaning of illness
in their lives.

CONSCIOUSNESS

A key factor in reempowering ourselves—in determining our purpose and intention, in reclaiming our own unique experience of

health and disease, and in making voluntary choices—is self-awareness or consciousness. Elgin (1981) described three levels of consciousness:

1. *Embedded consciousness,* in which we identify who we are with what we do. We think and feel from habit rather than from choice; we assume a social mask, which we protect and defend, and we hide our real self. The distinctive quality is self-forgetting.
2. *Self-reflective consciousness,* which involves a simultaneous awareness of details and an appreciation of the totality of life. The distinctive quality is self-remembering.
3. *Beyond self-reflective consciousness,* in which we tune into what we are experiencing in the moment such that boundaries between inner and outer selves dissolve.

Dossey (1984) discussed the experience of people who "go beyond" their illness. He referred to this stage as "immersion," which is comparable to Elgin's stage of "beyond self-reflective consciousness." "The distinctions between the knower and the known undergo a unification. These people experience a freedom from illness, even though they are afflicted by it and are immersed in it" (p. 61).

INCREASING SELF-AWARENESS

How do we move from automatic, habit-driven, embedded consciousness to self-reflective consciousness? The first thing to mention is that habits in and of themselves are not "bad." They serve a purpose in our survival by filtering out from our awareness certain repetitious behaviors, which can free up our awareness for other areas of focus, such as creativity. What generally happens, though, is that most of our thoughts, feelings, and actions become conditioned over time. We forget that many of these habits began as choices. We forget that we can change because we confuse what we "do" habitually with who we "are."

As well as clarifying our intention, voluntary change includes simply noticing, without judgment, what we are already doing, that is, attending to our current patterns of thought, feeling, and action. Bender (1989), who described her unique journey in her book *Plain and Simple,* addressed this aspect. "Before I could begin to simplify, I had to look at all the things that were filling up my life. Everything I was doing, everything I wanted to do, and everything I thought I had to do went into the symbolic pile—one large chaotic batch of desires crowding and bumping into each other" (p. 134). In noticing what we're doing, we begin to see the connection among the areas of our lives. We can then notice which behaviors are life-enhancing and which are life-blocking patterns.

We can "notice nonjudgmentally" on a feeling level by attending to our "felt sense" as we experience a pattern. "Sweeping the floor or doing the dishes is the outer form, the thing to which I attached myself in order to learn. What I had been looking for was the calm and focus I felt when I was with the Amish doing the dishes" (Bender, 1989, p. 145).

Out of our intellectual and experiential self-remembering, we may realize that certain habits need changing. Some habits may not seem to be personally harmful, but may be very harmful to the environment, or may be adversely affecting someone else's life-style. From a holistic point of view, when we harm others or the environment, whether intentionally or unintentionally, we harm ourselves.

Once we are aware of what we're doing, thinking, and feeling, we can decide what to release and what to retain. We begin to discriminate between beneficial and detrimental habits. "Part of the reason we do not try to simplify our lives is because we have come to believe that we need things that are in fact unnecessary. . . . When we appreciate the deep satisfaction of simple existence . . . we gain a new perspective on what in life are true benefits and what are actually liabilities that weigh heavily on our consciousness" (Cooper, 1992, p. 101).

As nurses, self-reflective consciousness involves asking ourselves questions pertaining to our nursing practice: What is health? What is disease? What is nursing? What is my objective as a nurse? How can I best practice nursing? How do I care for myself? What impact does this have on my care of others?

Newman's (1986) responses to some of these questions reflected her holistic point of view. "The patterns of interaction of person–environment constitute health. . . . pattern recognition is the essence of practice . . . what we sense in terms of pattern is a function of our own level of awareness, sensitivity to self, and point of view" (p. 18). Newman considered disease to be a clue that can facilitate understanding of one's own unique pattern in life.

The consciousness and intention with which we as nurses address our own experiences of disease will influence the manner in which we interact with our clients and with the imbalances of our larger environment. If we deny our illnesses, suppress or ignore symptoms and early warning signs, try merely to get rid of or quickly fix our disease, or label it as a meaningless nuisance in our lives, then these attitudes will be a part of our pattern of interaction with our clients. If we pay only lip service to the importance of illness as an aspect of health, then all our verbal and behavioral "caring" about our clients' illnesses will ring false and will not potentiate their healing. "We do not know how to savor health because we have lost the vital connections between health and illness . . . it is the felt organic connection to the world" (Dossey, 1985, p. 27).

The process of self-reflective consciousness is ongoing. It can be done at any time, but generally requires being in a quiet place and a relaxed state. Journaling may help to track the patterns. Just as larger worldview paradigms that were once cutting-edge become outdated, our own personal paradigms become outdated. Periodic reexamination is necessary. The extent and frequency of reexamination are up to the individual; there are no hard and fast rules. Tune into your intuitive knowing. The practice of self-reflective thinking will build upon itself. As your intentions clarify, new questions will emerge. This is the dynamic, evolving nature of living voluntarily. As Bender (1989) found, "Keeping the questions alive is important" (p. 137).

LIVING SIMPLY

Just as our intentions, whether voluntary or involuntary, guide and
determine our actions, so too the reverse is true: our actions reveal
our intentions. In other words, the initial focus in making changes
can be from the level of action rather than awareness. Each aspect
leads to the other. In her journey, Bender (1989) was first drawn
to the beauty of Amish quilts, which she sensed in some way related to her discomfort with her current life-style. Without clear intent or specific questions, she followed her intuition and went to
live for a period of time with the Amish. "When I started this journey, I didn't know my soul was starving. A tremendous need for
something led my spirit, guiding me in ways I often didn't understand, and didn't need to understand" (p. 142). Out of her intentional, daily participation in their simple life-style, a self-knowing
emerged. Out of her initial confusion and chaos, her questions and
answers emerged. Unconscious simplicity eventually became conscious simplicity that permeated her personal and professional life.
In terms of complexity theory, she reorganized her life at a higher
level of functioning.

> *To live with simplicity is to unburden our lives—to live*
> *more lightly, cleanly, aerodynamically. It means establish-*
> *ing a more direct, unpretentious, unencumbered relation-*
> *ship with all aspects of our lives. . . . Simplicity of living*
> *means meeting life face to face. It means confronting life*
> *clearly, without unnecessary distractions, without trying to*
> *soften the awesomeness of our existence or mask the deeper*
> *magnificence of life with pretentious, distracting, and un-*
> *necessary accumulations. It means being direct and honest*
> *in relationships of all kinds. It means taking life as it is—*
> *straight and unadulterated. (Elgin, 1981, p. 11)*

Simplicity is not about cutting back; it's about living in balance,
living more joyfully and creatively (Longacre, 1980). There are
many levels and paths, but no "perfect" way or path. You need to
look at the possibilities, assess which ones are best for you, test
them out through trial and error, see your mistakes as learning

experiences rather than judging them as failures, give yourself credit for the changes you make, and keep on trying. "My task is to simplify, and then go deeper, making a commitment to what remains . . . now I am ready to ask: 'Am I a successful human being, not only a success?'" (Bender, 1989, p. 145).

LEVELS OF CHANGE

Simplicity involves clearing up your outer physical environment. It also refers to simplifying your inner physical environment through self-care methods. Elgin (1981) presented a list of behaviors that included the following:

- Lowering overall consumption.
- Altering patterns of consumption in favor of products that are durable, easy to repair, and nonpolluting in their manufacture.
- Shifting diet away from highly processed foods.
- Pursuing work that directly contributes to the well-being of the world and simultaneously allows fuller use of individual creative capacities.
- Developing personal skills that contribute to greater self-reliance and reduce dependence on experts.
- Changing patterns of transportation and living closer to work. (p. 13)

Simplifying may also mean releasing worries and useless mental chatter that clog the mind, preventing positive and creative ideas from forming.

Our state of being, our mood, our interactions, our coping, our alertness, everything is related to the mind flow. . . . Almost all meditation technique is directed to the simplification of the mental process. Meditation practices can be enhanced if we structure the external process of living in simple terms. . . . The more simply we organize our lives, the more rewarding we will find our inner work. (Cooper, 1992, p. 101)

Emotional simplicity may involve letting go of old emotional baggage that distracts you from enjoying the present. In relationships, it may include saying what you mean directly, rather than talking around difficult issues. Financially, it may mean cleaning up old debts and simplifying your budget.

For more ideas on specific changes you can test out, there are books on the market that suggest, for example: reducing clutter, time management, making dietary changes to eat lower on the food chain, clearing out unwanted thoughts and emotions, assessing environmental toxins in your home and workplace, identifying healthy alternatives, and simple self-care behaviors at work. *Wellness: Small Changes You Can Use to Make a Big Difference* (Ryan & Travis, 1991) and *50 Simple Things You Can Do to Save the Earth* (Earthworks Group, 1991) are two good books to start with. Dossey (1985) discusses nursing self-care and patient-care techniques in her article, "Holistic Nursing: How to Make It Work for You."

BENEFITS OF VOLUNTARY SIMPLICITY

To begin any one of these new behaviors from square one may mean a large initial investment of time, but in the long run, as the new behavior becomes a healthier habit, the investment will more than pay for itself, in ways you may not expect. Moving in the direction of voluntary simplicity will balance out the "things" in your life with the "meaning" in your life, both professionally and personally. You may find yourself feeling healthier, having closer relationships with family, friends, and neighbors. You may find a creative side of yourself you didn't know existed.

In your nursing work, benefits may translate into greater job satisfaction, perhaps even a long-needed job change. You'll find that you can be more available to your clients by ridding yourself of unnecessarily cluttering mental and emotional distractions; you may help clients to see their illnesses in a different way that emphasizes quality of life and promotes healthier coping mechanisms as a result. You'll be able to convey this from your own experience rather than just giving textbook information. Your words will have greater impact because you'll be living them. You'll know what it takes to make life-style changes. You'll see and help clients to see the possibilities for well-being that exist even within their experience of illness.

If, as Dossey (1984) says, health is an "experience," not just a static event or future goal, then you'll be modeling this to your clients just by freeing yourself up to be present to your own living experience, as well as present to whatever your client is experiencing in that moment. This in itself is healing. Through the property of resonance, you'll be a part of a healing environment with your clients.

Voluntary simplicity will also promote a greater internal strength, placing you in a better position to protect yourself from imbalances you might encounter in your work. You may take fewer sick days when formerly you had frequently succumbed to illnesses, or you may find that you need to take more time for yourself instead of pushing yourself to work no matter what. You'll assess the level of health or toxicity in your environments, identifying physical toxins and nonphysical toxins (for example, toxic relationships).

Building a support system for this work is beneficial. It might be of help to find or form a group of supportive individuals who are also interested in simplifying their lives in conscious, deliberate, and creative ways. Let your family know of your intention and elicit their support. If they are not supportive, don't clutter up your life by worrying about it. Do what you can independently, and find supportive people outside of your family. Cut out articles about other people who are making similar changes, and keep a support notebook. Keep a journal of your journey on this path. Again, self-awareness and self-responsibility are aspects of nurturing yourself.

SUMMARY

Voluntary simplicity is a holistic, ecological framework for dealing with the necessary complexities of personal, professional, and planetary life. As many nursing theorists indicate, each of these aspects affects the others, so it is imperative that we attend to the choices we make. In choosing to simplify our lives, we eliminate unnecessary complexities produced by living in the more-is-better mode. We create more space and time for a balance of being and doing, and we find that we actually have more with less. As our self-awareness increases, we become more connected with our lived experience, and we are present to assist our clients in dealing with their lived experience.

The changes we make toward healthier, healing environments in both our personal lives and our nursing profession will, in turn, support us as we move with joy and creativity through our life's natural cycles.

PERSONAL STATEMENT

At the age of 17, a family camping trip to Yellowstone began my love affair with nature. It was an eye-opener after 17 years spent primarily in the city of Chicago. During the next four years of nursing school, I took off every summer to visit a national park, where I learned wilderness backpacking and hiking. Armed with a nursing degree, I moved to Alaska for three years and lived close to the elements and in the midst of pristine beauty. During these experiences, I befriended people whose lives integrated their environmental awareness with a sense of responsibility for their own health. This was new for me. Although I had a great deal of knowledge about disease, I started to realize that I didn't know much about health, especially my own health. As my consciousness expanded to incorporate holistic principles, I began to see the discrepancies between my beliefs about health and my life-style, between the health care system within which I practiced nursing, and the effects of my beliefs and practices on the local and global environment.

I was inspired to return to school in order to ground my awareness in the structure of a graduate program in holistic health. I have returned to Chicago, where I now implement my learnings in a private practice in wellness counseling. I am a member of a number of environmental groups, and recently was on the planning committee for the first "urban" Great Lakes Bioregional Congress. I have participated in prairie restoration work, a wonderful way to do hands-on environmental healing work. I also work at a hospital as a psychiatric nurse and I have joined the Recycling Committee. In whatever I do, I strive to practice what I preach: being present in the moment with intentionality, maintaining awareness of my oneness with the environment, and taking responsibility for my choices.

REFERENCES

American Heritage Dictionary of the English Language. (1970). New York: Houghton Mifflin.

Bender, S. (1989). *Plain and simple: A woman's journey to the Amish.* New York: Harper & Row.

Burkhardt, M. (1985). Nursing, health and wholeness. *Journal of Holistic Nursing, 3*(1), 35–36.

Cooper, D. (1992). *Silence, simplicity, solitude: A guide for spiritual retreat.* New York: Belltower.

Davidson, A., & Ray, M. (1991). Studying the human–environment phenomenon using the science of complexity. *Advances in Nursing Science, 14*(2), 73–87.

Dossey, B. (1985). Holistic nursing: How to make it work for you. *Journal of Holistic Nursing, 1*(1), 32–36.

Dossey, L. (1984). *Beyond illness: Discovering the experience of health.* Boston: Shambhala.

Earthworks Group, The. (1991). *50 simple things you can do to save the earth.* Berkeley, CA: Earth Works Press.

Elgin, D. (1981). *Voluntary simplicity: An ecological life-style that promotes personal and social renewal.* New York; Bantam.

Gaut, D. (1993). Caring: A vision of wholeness for nursing. *Journal of Holistic Nursing, 2*(2), 164–171.

Gregg, R. (1936, August). Voluntary simplicity. *Visva-Bharati Quarterly.*

Longacre, D. (1980). *Living more with less.* Scottsdale, AZ: Herald Press.

Newman, M. (1986). *Health as expanding consciousness.* St. Louis: Mosby.

Newman, M. (1990). Shifting to higher consciousness. In M. Parker (Ed.), *Nursing theories in practice.* New York: National League for Nursing.

Rogers, M. (1970). *An introduction to the theoretical basis of nursing.* Philadelphia: Davis.

Ryan, R., & Travis, J. (1991). *Wellness: Small changes you can use to make a big difference.* Berkeley, CA: Ten Speed Press.

Watson, J. (1988). New dimensions of human caring theory. *Nursing Science Quarterly, 1*(4): 175–181.

In the Gloom of the Environmental Crisis, Can Nurses Afford to Dwell in Hope and Be Defined by the Past?

Dianne Lacroix

INTRODUCTION

This chapter discusses the urgent need for nursing professionals to define the nature of their commitment toward the paradigm shift necessary to resolve the environmental crisis. Powerful and innovative strategies, comparable to the introduction of the nursing process, need to be initiated to promote ecologically sustainable life-styles and health care delivery systems. By the very nature of their profession, nurses are in an optimal position to assist in the understanding of the meaning of change and the process necessary for an ecological perspective of health. Nurses can participate in the environmental movement by supporting a professional, holistic, multidisciplinary, and transcultural approach to health care and health promotion. This chapter demonstrates how an expressive orientation to nursing care, within the framework of the educational model of health care, can provide the means to transcend the constraints of the biomedical model that perpetuate a dissociation from the natural environment. The environmental crisis will be a unique opportunity to express the essence of nursing through a collective ecological self, if nurses unite globally to invent a sustainable future.

> *My son, my daughter, and I were standing in silence, listening to the music, bathing in the ecstasy that emerges as one experiences the Light and Sound Spectacular at the Epcot Center in Disney World, Florida. In the midst of colorful laser beams, fireworks, light pictures, water fountains, and the successive illumination of the countries' pavilions, which transforms the World Showcase Lagoon into shimmering scenes, my nine-year-old daughter asked: "Mom, are fireworks bad for the environment?"*

The global economic and environmental crises of the 1990s are challenging our worldviews on health, education, and the knowledge to promote sustainable life-styles and well-being. These crises have accelerated the rate of change in the health care system with profound ramifications in all domains of professional education and practice. Thus, the new ecological–economic paradigm (Ehrlich & Ehrlich, 1992) will provide the greatest challenge for nurses to define and assert their commitment to universal well-being of the present and future generations, and the ecosystems that support health. It has become more crucial than ever to reflect on the subjective and collective meaning of change, and to address the need for visionary leadership. We, as nurses, must explore the frameworks that could provide guidelines and a sense of direction for healing the planet.

In this chapter, I explore why it is urgent that nurses define the nature of their commitment to the changes necessary toward ecological harmony and balance. Although some nurses are responding globally to a call to become informed, to lighten their own impact on the biosphere, and to be politically engaged (Ehrlich & Ehrlich, 1992), will the profession of nursing use the opportunity of a paradigm shift for soul searching, for taking stock, and for looking ahead? Innovative solutions must be implemented urgently; the deterioration of the environment cannot wait for nurses to define their commitment and approach. By the very intimate nature of nursing, nurses are placed in an optimal position to understand and promote a conceptualization of the deep changes necessary to effect sustainability.

I also highlight how an ecological approach to health challenges the very essence of nursing and a deeper understanding of the meaning of a holistic, multidisciplinary, professional, and transcultural approach to nursing care. I argue that the changes toward an ecological view of health cannot be effected within the constraints of the biomedical model; alternate models of health care that have more affinity with the key themes of successful improvement and an ecological view of the world must be supported. The principles of an expressive orientation to nursing care (Lacroix, 1991; Stanton, 1986; Wolfe, 1982), such as self-care and mutual goal setting, need to be promoted if nurses are to remain the nucleus of the health care system and the patient's advocate for holistic health and harmony with the natural environment. What key questions must we address, then, subjectively and collectively, toward the development of a collective and universal ecological self?

THE NATURE OF A NURSE'S COMMITMENT

If the notion of a Kuhnian paradigm shift (Kuhn, 1970) is accepted, then the very nature of a revolution in beliefs, values, frames of reference, and evaluation can only exacerbate the nursing profession's struggle to define its essence. Baume (1992), in describing the rapid rate of change in the health care system, suggested that "it is likely that we are moving through a period of Kuhnian scientific revolution, in the process from one stable paradigm to another. What the new paradigm is we can not yet see clearly. What is apparent is that the old paradigm is finished and inadequate" (p. 4). The period of a paradigm shift, with its associated uncertainties, debates, and conflicts, can provide the opportunity for defining an ecological view of health by addressing some deep questions and conflicts. Among these are:

- Will the profession of nursing survive the rapid rate of change and strongly articulate its essence through the turmoils of a paradigm shift? Will nurses define their commitment to universal well-being in terms of its past history of domination, and continue to "willingly [participate] in coattailing the medical profession?" (Beaumont, 1987, p. 48)
- Will nurses' commitment to universal well-being and holistic care prove to be just a plethora of words?

Some nurses and nursing organizations have understood that we cannot afford to ignore the call for action in the hope that the problems will go away. From the Declaration of Alma-Ata on Primary Health Care in 1978, and the First International Conference on Health Promotion in Industrialized Countries, in 1986, nurses made formal and informal contributions to global sustainable health care. Worldwide concern for health and the environment led to a series of important global gatherings to consider the issues (see Table 15–1).

The Ottawa Charter for Health Promotion (1986, p. 5) formally acknowledges that "caring, holism and ecology are essential issues in developing strategies for health promotion" and for moving into the future. The Adelaide Recommendations led the Australian Nursing Federation to adopt a 12-point Green Care Plan (1990) and to release, in January 1993, a Health Policy Document that stresses that "the environment suffers no damage as the result of the operations of the health industry" (Australian Nursing Federation, 1993). The International Council of Nurses (1991b) declared, in a health and ecology statement, that "nurses worldwide, as key health professionals, are in a unique position to act as constructive agents of change." The contribution to environmental awareness by Nursing the Environment, the special interest group of the Australian Nursing Federation (Victoria), was formally acknowledged in a statement of the Office of the Status of Women

**Table 15–1 Summary of Major Events
Leading to the Summit in June 1992**

Event	Year and Country/Sponsor	Outcome
30th World Health Assembly	1977, World Health Organization	Health for All by the Year 2000
International Conference on Primary Health Care	1978, Alma-Ata, USSR	Declaration of Alma-Ata on Primary Health Care
First International Conference on Health Promotion in Industrialized Countries	1986, Ottawa, Canada	Ottawa Charter for Health Promotion
Meeting for the United Nations Environment Program	1987, Montreal, Canada	Montreal Protocol
World Commission on Health and Environment	1987, United Nations	Our Common Future (Bruntland Report)
Healthy Public Policy Conference	1988, Adelaide, Australia	Adelaide Recommendations
Call for Action: Health Promotion in Developing Countries	1989, Geneva, Switzerland	International Network of Health-Promoting Hospitals
Conference on Supportive Environments for Health	1991, Sundsvall, Sweden	Sundsvall Statement
WHO Business Meeting	1991, Budapest, Hungary	Budapest Declaration
UNCED, Earth Summit, Indigenous People's Forum	1992, Rio de Janeiro, Brazil	Agenda 21; Earth Charter; Rio Declaration

(1992, p. 9), prepared for the United Nations Conference in Rio de Janeiro. Nursing the Environment provided a forum for active debate and exploration of the links between health and ecology at the first Australian Conference in March 1993 (Lucas & Lacroix, 1993). The activities of this green professional organization assist nurses in expressing a definite political stand (Nursing the Environment, 1990).

Although the International Council of Nurses recognizes and acknowledges the vital role that nurses can play in finding solutions to environmental degradation at the global level (International

Council of Nurses, 1991a, 1991b), the Council did not formally represent the profession of nursing at the most important historical event for sustainability, in Rio de Janeiro, in June 1992 (International Council of Nurses, personal communication, 1993). We, as nurses and as key health professionals, have the obligation to understand the implications of the major commitments to health as expressed in these documents since 1977, and to monitor and ensure the implementations of these recommendations, however difficult, in times of economic crises. The governments are now accountable for the implementation of the treaties on biodiversity and global warming that were signed in June 1992: the Rio Declaration, the Earth Charter, and Agenda 21.

In Australia, the active promotion of sustainable life-styles and health care systems has become more difficult in the midst of an economic crisis. Recent research by a pollster (Murphy, 1993, p. 36) during the national election campaign in early 1993 indicated a shift in thinking and values. The environment is "seen by some as an '80s issue. The recession has made the ecological issues appear to be expensive and politically expendable." This shift in values translates into a move from the green issues of the 1980s to what Environment Minister Kelly calls the "brown issues": industrial waste, sewage, and chemicals. Ultimately, these will demand more perseverance and efforts to implement strategies such as the Australian Nursing Federation's 12-point Green Care Plan within individual workplaces (Australian Nursing Federation, 1990). The nurses' vital role in raising awareness of ecological issues among health care professionals and reducing the environmental impact of the health care system is therefore crucial. Health care professional groups, such as the Australian Medical Association, have no position statement on environmental issues (Australian Medical Association, 1992).

Although Australian nurses are leading the way in health and ecology (Nurses take lead . . . , 1992, December), it has taken 20 years for nurses to formally acknowledge their responsibility toward the environment. Many nurses practicing in the 1970s and 1980s have now come to understand how unaware and uninformed they are of the environmental impact of the health care system. Yet, nursing authors such as Levine were questioning the links between health and the deterioration of the environment in the early 1970s. Levine (1971, p. 254) described the links between holism and an ecological approach to health, and expressed a deep concern for the safety of future generations:

> *And while dualism was perpetuated in the individual, the relationship of the individual to his wider environments was dissociated into the specious nature-nurture argument. It has come as something of a cultural and political shock that technologic progress has so altered the biosphere as to threaten seriously the future safety of human life. Analytical, dualistic dominance in scientific thought has so immuned [the] twentieth century from realistic awareness of the threat of altered environments that even this issue is debated, disputed, and disclaimed, and meanwhile, the degradation of all living things moves inexorably onward.*

Some nurses have taken two decades to understand the insights of theorists such as Levine, and to start addressing the dichotomies of health promotion in an environment that inhibits or constrains their efforts toward sustainable life-styles and health care. Nurses are constantly experiencing the implications of polluted water and air, and unhealthy soil, such as the known effect of lead pollution on children's health, while caring for their patients, families, and communities. Chopoorian referred to the dichotomy of the two worlds of nursing—the one we teach about and the one that is—and described nurses as the witnesses of the everyday realities of the links between health and the total environment:

> *More and more every day, we observe forces that work against people's health and well-being; unemployment and underemployment, lack of adequate housing, lack of access to health services, poverty, racism, sexism, pollution of the environment, production of hazardous materials, and opportunistic foreign and military policies which drain resources for domestic programs and have produced a federal deficit unparalleled in our history. (Chopoorian, 1990, p. 21)*

THE MEANING OF CHANGE

A call for action, despite uncertainties, doubts, and lack of a definite sense of direction, is very evident in recommendations for healing the planet. Baume (1992, p. 4) stated, in relation to the changes in the health care system: "We are likely to get just one opportunity to create and to implement the new paradigm, whether the period of 'revolution' is short or long. If we can give the commitment with whatever wisdom we possess it is likely to be more successful than if we stand aloof or apart." Whatever wisdom we possess can be drawn from reflections on the collective and subjective meaning of change that nurses experience constantly in their practice. Change is a recurrent theme in nursing practice and nursing education, as nurses help patients cope with imposed and different life-styles. A conceptualization of human responses to change could be drawn from each individual nurse's perceptions of the meaning of transition toward a viable future. If nurses took the opportunity to reflect on the meaning of change, to share their perceptions and their experiences in order to validate one another's thoughts and knowledge, a conceptualization could be drawn from their practical knowledge and skills. Nurses can be supported in learning to appreciate the contribution they can make toward an ecological view of health and a holistic perspective of human responses to transition and a cultural revolution.

Nurses, as a professional community, can foster the understanding of the collective meaning of change. A dynamic and vivid picture of the change process, within the framework of the key themes of successful improvement in education (Fullan & Stiegelbauer, 1991), would promote a sound approach and instill more confidence of success. The six interrelated themes of successful changes in education, as identified by Fullan and Stiegelbauer (1991, pp. 81-82), are: (1) vision building, (2) evolutionary planning and development, (3) initiative taking and empowerment, (4) monitoring and problem coping, (5) staff development and resource assistance, and (6) restructuring.

Nursing leaders, authors, educators, and theorists have therefore an extremely important role in articulating an ecological vision of nursing and fostering active participation in the change process by all nurses. The dynamic interactions of the processes of vision building, active participation, and involvement by all health care professionals in all domains must be promoted for the implementation of innovative and creative solutions to the environmental crisis. As Boyce (1991, p. 147) stated: "The current flirtation of health administrators with organizational restructuring has major implications for the working environment of all health workers. However, those with low levels of political organization and access to decision-making apparatus are least likely to mount effective responses."

Through the very intimate nature of nursing and its role within the health care system, nurses occupy an optimal position to understand and promote the subjective meaning of change. Nurses have the unique opportunity of enabling the support necessary for all the small steps toward a life-style conducive to health and sustainability. As Fullan and Stiegelbauer (1991, p. 55) pointed out, "[T]he innovative paradigm, which in effect traces the development and implementation of formally initiated innovations, is biased because it misses the thousands of small innovations that individual and small groups of teachers engage in every day." A nursing conceptualization of successful and valued changes through support, encouragement, and active participation, implemented in the everyday practices of nurses, could foster an understanding of the change process and an awareness of the possible outcomes. The pressure for different ways of being can raise uncertainties and inhibit all efforts toward change:

> *Change can be very deep, striking at the core of learned skills and beliefs and conceptions of education, creating doubts about purposes, sense of competence, and self-concept. If these problems are ignored or glossed over, superficial change will occur at best; at worst, people will retreat into a self-protective cocoon, unreflectively rejecting all proposed changes. Even changes that do not seem to be complex to their promoter may raise numerous doubts and uncertainties on the part of those not familiar with them. (Fullan & Stiegelbauer, 1991, p. 45)*

THE NEED FOR A HOLISTIC, PROFESSIONAL, MULTIDISCIPLINARY, AND TRANSCULTURAL APPROACH TO HEALTH CARE

A conceptualization of change toward an ecological view of health is also congruent with a defined holistic approach and an "emphasis or value of the whole but with consideration of discrete parts that are interrelated" (Wheeler & Chinn, 1991, p. 199). A holistic and ecological approach "attempts to emphasize the interaction between the mind, body and spirit that constitutes health, but also relates health to the wider concept of an ecosystem that strives for balance" (Kickbusch, 1989, p. 5). Boyden (1980, p. 625) defined the wider concept as three levels of reality relating to human health and well-being:

Level 1—the biopsychic state of individuals or groups of individuals;

Level 2—the life conditions of individuals or groups of individuals;

Level 3—the total environment.

At these three levels of health, Boyden referred to two categories of variables relevant to human health and well-being: (1) tangible and (2) intangible, with some variables intermediate in their classification. The tangible variables, such as blood pressure or amount of subcutaneous fat, are relatively easy to measure and describe. The intangible variables are those that "cannot be quantified and . . . are difficult to describe in precise terms" (Boyden, 1980, p. 627); they "include the individual's knowledge, values, wants, and his or her mental state, mood, and such feelings as a sense of personal involvement, of comradeship, of security, of belonging, of disappointment or frustration."

It is important to reflect on the implications of the "intangibility" of some health variables for nursing care. As Boyden pointed out, humans innately find dealing with the tangibles much easier and more acceptable; they are concrete and easy to describe. It calls for a "special intellectual effort" to study the intangible variables, and we must therefore "work to develop ways and means which will help us to come to grips with them, to identify them, to communicate effectively about them, and to ensure that they are properly taken into account in our analysis of human situations and in our planning for the future" (Boyden, 1980, p. 629). Once again, the very intimate nature of nursing care places nurses in a special position to contribute to the promotion of an understanding of the role that the intangibles play in human health and well-being.

The inclusion of intangible variables in the planning of a viable future and the healing of the planet calls for a true multidisciplinary approach to health care. As Kickbusch (1989, p. 11) stated, "Public health needs to rise above petty professional squabbles over specialized fields of intervention to a generalist and policy-based concern for the health of populations, which can no longer be separated from the social mechanisms that produce risks to health." Nurses now work with other professionals as valuable and indispensable members on environmental committees, such as waste management, in the hospital and community setting. Nurses are often at the forefront of changes, as the largest group of health professionals and consumers of health care products that have a large and negative impact on the environment.

The challenge of a true multidisciplinary approach to health care and problem solving can also be addressed by initiatives such as those taken by the School of Health, University of Newcastle, Australia (Graham & Honari, 1990). Through education, the School of Health is reinforcing the view that a transdisciplinary approach to the examination of health problems is vital for the development of a human ecological perspective. The core health curriculum for all undergraduate health professionals provides a model for future developments. The nursing profession will naturally express some concerns in losing its identity in a transdisciplinary approach to education and a multidisciplinary approach to health. However, it is important to value a transdisciplinary approach to health education as an opportunity to experience the intraprofessional differences and the special contribution that nursing can make toward an ecological approach. Contrasts in professionals' views and qualities are essential for the creation of innovative solutions to the environmental crisis. A strong essence can only emerge through the process of differentiation in a divergent and pluralistic structure (Teilhard de Chardin, 1959). As Dinesen (1960, p. 408) described, unity of contrasts is essential for creative problem solving:

> *In order to form and make a Unity, in particular a creative Unity, the individual components must needs be of different nature, they should even be in a sense contrasts. Two homogenous units will never be capable of forming a whole. . . . A hook and an eye are a Unity, a fastening; but with two hooks you can do nothing. A right-hand glove with its contrast the left-hand glove makes up a whole, a pair of gloves; but two right-hand gloves you throw away. A number of perfectly similar objects do not make up a whole.*

THE CONSTRAINTS OF THE
BIOMEDICAL MODEL OF CARE

A holistic and ecological approach cannot be promoted by adhering strictly to the philosophy of the biomedical model of health care, with its emphasis on curing and the mind–body dichotomy based on the Cartesian concept of the person (Capra, 1982). An understanding of the need for a cultural revolution that transcends the shortcomings of this biomedical model involves the articulation of alternate views, without the replacement of one dogma with another. Support for alternative ways of being can be initiated through the integration of different philosophies of care, such as the educational model of health care (Bartlett, 1987), with its emphasis on holism, self-responsibility, and care. The educational model provides a framework to promote the six successful themes of improvement in education (Fullan & Stiegelbauer, 1991), with emphasis on active participation and problem coping. The philosophy of the educational model is congruent with an expressive orientation to nursing care (Lacroix, 1991). A holistic and ecological concept of health will require active participation by all recipients of care, and the fostering of self-responsibility. "As a society we tend to use medical diagnosis as a cover-up of social problems" (Capra, 1982, p. 165), and some patients will naturally resist the changes toward alternate models of care because they object to examining their life-styles and taking responsibility for their well-being and their impact on the biosphere.

Nursing, therefore, plays a vital role in creating supportive theoretical models of health care that promote a patient-centered and holistic approach, and value information as therapeutic, universal health and self-care. An ecological perspective of health care requires more than an acknowledgment of the limitations of the biomedical model, because it is more than a model, as Capra (1982, p. 164) described: "Among the medical profession it has acquired the status of a dogma, and for the general public it is inextricably linked to the common cultural belief system. To go beyond it will require nothing less than a profound cultural revolution." Although some nurses have experienced and perceived the constraints of the biomedical model, more efforts are needed to continue the expansion of the nurses' role as holistic healers and health educators with a transcultural perspective. The understanding of the role of culture is important in distinguishing true universal health needs (Boyden, Dovers, & Shirlow, 1990) from culturally defined human wants.

A professional approach to patient education reflects an understanding of the principles of an expressive and/or nonexpressive orientation to nursing care (Stanton, 1986; Wolfe, 1982). A literature review (Lacroix, 1991) on the patient education role in nursing described the link between the approach of the biomedical model of health care to a nonexpressive orientation to nursing care, and that of the educational model to an expressive orientation. The same literature review on patient education (Lacroix, 1991) also highlighted a lack of consensus on the goals of patient teaching: compliance and/or self-care. Some nursing authors believe that the term compliance, with its authoritarian overtones of obedience and conformity, has become somewhat obsolete. Other nursing authors use the two terms as if they are interchangeable and compatible with the nursing goals of self-care and an equitable relationship of teacher/learner. The unresolved question of the aims of patient education needs to be addressed for a clearer understanding and affirmation of nursing's goals. Nursing's contribution to the resolution of the environmental crisis may provide a strong impetus toward evaluating whether nursing is supporting the goal of curing, thus reflecting a medical dominance, or the goal of caring as an expression of the essence of nursing.

UNITY IN COLLECTIVE ECOLOGICAL SELF

Through the fulfillment of our ecological responsibilities, different kinds of knowing and of being in nursing will be fully explored and expressed. As Case (1992, p. 18) suggested, "It is our capacity to know, to love and to heal that gives us ethical and ecological responsibilities." A collective ecological self could be expressed in nursing by providing a deeper understanding of what nurses *really want* for themselves, for their patients, and for future generations, and by addressing four basic questions (Graham & Honari, 1990) at the universal level:

1. What can I know?
2. Where do I stand?
3. What ought I do?
4. What can I hope?

To explore there four basic questions, an equal emphasis and value of the four fundamental patterns of knowing in nursing, as identified by Carper (1978)—empirics, ethics, personal, and esthetics—is essential in nursing education, practice, and research. A holistic and ecological approach to knowing would give equal value to different ways of understanding the tangible and intangible variables of health and well-being of humans and the biosphere at the three levels of reality (Boyden, 1980). Such an approach values equally the rational and logic, associated with the masculine way of knowing, and intuition and synthesis, associated with the feminine way. Conflicts resolved by the masculine process of domination have resulted in technical and chemical wars with vast damages to the ecosystems. An ecological approach must therefore promote the feminist process (Wheeler & Chinn, 1991) of consensus formation toward a peaceful, harmonious, and dynamic coexistence of diverse ways of being. Different ways of knowing promotes diverse ways of being; the harmonious mind–body–soul of the individual will be connected with the environment and each other individual.

The period of intense debating and questioning associated with a paradigm shift and with the change process necessary for the healing of the planet will provide the impetus for all nurses to reflect on the meaning and the implications of what they really want, more than anything, for self, family, peers, community, patients/clients. Dyer (1985) asked the same questions from a parent's perspective and proposed these collective parental goals for our children's future: I want my children to value themselves, to be risk-takers, to be self-reliant, to be free from stress and anxiety, to have peaceful lives, to celebrate their present moments, to experience a lifetime of wellness, to be creative, to fulfill their higher needs, and to feel a sense of purpose. Would nurses find similar answers if they reflected on the same fundamental questions, subjectively and collectively, at the universal level? If nurses were to actively question what they really want in the future, for themselves and their patients, powerful and articulated visions could provide the power of one voice, "the power of *one*—one idea, one heart, one mind, one plan, one determination" (Courtenay, 1989, p. 124). Basic nursing goals cannot be attained globally if fresh air, clean water, and healthy soils are not available to meet the universal health needs of humans and ecosystems.

POSTSCRIPT OF MARCH 1994

A whole year of thinking, reflecting, writing, networking, researching, and parenting has gone by since I attended the International Conference. The events of 1993 contributed to a deepening of my understanding and my theoretical sensitivity. The special interest group of the Australian Nursing Federation, Nursing the

Environment, achieved national status in September 1993. In the same month, our Professor of Nursing at La Trobe University, Judy Parker, offered to hold the position of President and to actively support the efforts and the activities of Nursing the Environment. We, as members of the Executive, are most grateful to have the assistance of such a visionary leader of nursing.

These events have reaffirmed for me the vital role that nurses, as predominantly females in a caring profession, can play in the raising of ecological awareness. We are in a most powerful position to promote the awareness of the need to change our Western values to those more conducive to living in harmony and balance with healthy ecosystems and with each other. As David Susuki pointed out (1993, p. 194), "Women are the critical element in the environmental movement both for their point of view and their lack of vested interests in the current power structures." An innate sensitivity associated with feminine ways of knowing can support the promotion of understanding and conceptualization of the intangibles of health and the intangibles of knowing, such as wisdom. A holistic vision of a healthy future incorporates the tangibles and the intangibles, the masculine and the feminine, the yin and the yang in harmony and balance, as to express a broad vision for the full solution to environmental problems, and to reflect the interconnectedness of life (Shepherd, 1993). Can we, as nurses, practitioners, academics, researchers, and teachers, rise to the challenge before it is too late, or will we be accused of compartmentalized thinking by the next generations?

PERSONAL STATEMENT

In March 1990, I returned to a university in Melbourne, Australia, to complete postgraduate studies. I found some entirely new concepts fascinating, as described by Professor Judy Parker in the unit of the History and Philosophy of Nursing. I particularly developed a keen interest in the philosophies of deep ecology and ecofeminism. Through discussion, I could identify some major sources of ethical conflicts for nurses, such as the protection of elephants and/or the protection of the poachers who had become victims of a conservation program. I could only describe the short-term implications for nursing from a shallow environmental perspective.

In 1992, I joined a Green Nursing support group, Nursing the Environment, a special interest group of the Victorian Branch of the Australian Nursing Federation. I became a member of the steering committee for the first National Health and Ecology Conference (March 1993) in Melbourne, Victoria. Through Nursing the Environment, I met many dedicated and informed nurses, from the various domains of nursing, who give their time and skills on a voluntary basis to promote ecological awareness. In September 1992, I accepted the position of assistant secretary, to support the aims and objectives of this special interest group at a political level. The enthusiasm of the members of Nursing the Environment, and the visionary leadership of Helen Lucas, the Secretary, inspired me to continue to explore the implications of an ecological approach to nursing at the Master's level in 1992. I am presently completing a study at La Trobe University, investigating the visions of a healthy future held by eight nurses active in the promotion of the links between health and ecology.

Through my studies and my activities as a member of Nursing the Environment, I became acutely aware of the need for ecologically sensitive life-styles, and of my personal and professional responsibilities toward future generations. Every day, I try to implement the principles of voluntary simplicity as discussed in Florida in March 1993 in the forum facilitated by Kathleen Musker (1993). I am fully aware that it is most necessary for my children's healthy future that they are totally sensitive to the needs of the planet and take the necessary steps toward wise ways of knowing.

REFERENCES

Australian Medical Association. (1992). Letter from P. S. Wilkins to D. Lacroix. *The Australian Nurses Journal, 22*(8), 21.

Australian Nursing Federation. (1990). Australian Nursing Federation Policy Statements, *The Australian Nurses Journal, 19*(10), 21.

Australian Nursing Federation. (1993). Health Policy, *The Australian Nurses Journal, 22*(7), 6–11.

Bartlett, E. (1987). The educational model of health care. *Canadian Nurse, 83*(9), 3.

Baume, P. (1992, October). Political agendas and restructuring of health services in Australia. *Proceedings of the Multidisciplinary Conference on Managing Matters in Health Care.* Melbourne, Australia: Department of Nursing, La Trobe University.

Beaumont, M. K. (1987). The nursing struggle. *The Australian Nurses Journal, 17*(3), 48–51.

Boyce, R. A. (1991). Hospital restructuring—the implications for allied health professions. *Australian Health Review, 14*(2), 147–154.

Boyden, S. (1980). The need for an holistic approach to human health and well-being. In N. F. Stanley & R. A. Joske (Eds.), *Changing disease patterns and human behaviour* (pp. 621–644). Sydney: Academic Press.

Boyden, S., Dovers, S., & Shirlow, M. (1990). *Our biosphere under threat: Ecological realities and Australia's opportunities.* Melbourne: Oxford University Press.

Capra, F. (1982). *The turning point: Science, society and the rising culture.* London: Flamingo.

Carper, B. A. (1978). Fundamental patterns of knowing in nursing. *Advances in Nursing Science, 1*(1), 13–23.

Case, J. M. (1992). The biosphere and the healing arts. *Holistic Nursing Practice, 6*(4), 10–19.

Chopoorian, T. J. (1990). The two worlds of nursing: The one we teach about, the one that is. In National League for Nursing, *Curriculum Revolution: Redefining the Student-Teacher Relationship* (pp. 21–36). New York: National League for Nursing.

Courtenay, B. (1989). *The power of one.* Australia: Mandarin.

Dinesen, I. (1960). *Shadows on the grass.* New York: Vintage Books.

Dyer, W. W. (1985). *What do you really want for your children?* New York: Avon Books.

Ehrlich, P. R., & Ehrlich, A. H. (1992). *Healing the planet: Strategies for resolving the environmental crisis.* Australia: Surrey Beatty & Sons.

Fullan, M. G., & Stiegelbauer, S. (1991). *The new meaning of educational change.* New York: Teachers College, Columbia University.

Graham, J., & Honari, M. (1990). Human ecology and health advancement: The Newcastle experience and implications. *Journal of Human Ecology, 2*(1/2), 197–215.

International Council of Nurses. (1991a, July). *Nurses commit them-selves to quest for a sustainable future.* News Release No. 4. Geneva, Switzerland.

International Council of Nurses. (1991b, June). *The nurse and the environmental issues.* Position statement. Geneva, Switzerland.

International Council of Nurses. (1993, July). Personal communication from ICN to D. Lacroix. Geneva, Switzerland.

Kickbusch, I. (1989). Good planets are hard to find. *World Health Cities Paper No. 5.* Copenhagen: FADL.

Kuhn, T. (1970). *The structure of scientific revolutions* (2nd ed.). Chicago: University of Chicago Press.

Lacroix, D. (1991). *A pilot survey of nurses' attitudes towards the nurse-patient relationship in the teaching situation within a hospital setting.* Unpublished preliminary Master's thesis, La Trobe University, Lincoln School of Health Sciences, Department of Nursing, Melbourne, Australia.

Levine, M. E. (1971). Holistic nursing. *Nursing Clinics of North America, 6*(2), 253-264.

Lucas, H., & Lacroix, D. (1993). Spinning the web: Taking health and ecology from the margin into the mainstream. *The Australian Nurses Journal, 22*(10), 6-9.

Murphy, D. (1993). 93 Election: A paler shade of green. *Australian Time, 93*(9), 36.

Musker, K. (1993). *Promoting an ecological lifestyle through voluntary simplicity.* Presentation conference on expressions of caring in nursing: Exploring our environmental connections. See Chapter 14, this volume.

Nurses take lead on ecology and health. (1992, December). *Better Health Briefing, 2*(1), 12.

Nursing the Environment. (1990). *Statement of purpose/Aims and objectives.* Melbourne, Australia: Australian Nursing Federation.

Office of the Status of Women (Department of the Prime Minister and Cabinet). (1992). *Women and the environment.* Canberra, Australia: Commonwealth Government Publishing.

Ottawa Charter for Health Promotion. (1986). International Conference on Health Promotion. Ottawa, Canada: World Health Organization, Health and Welfare, Canada, & Canadian Public Association.

Shepherd, L. J. (1993). *Lifting the veil: The feminine face of science.* Boston: Shambhala.

Stanton, P. (1986). Nurses' attitudes toward nurse–patient interaction in the patient-teaching situation. *Nursing Success Today, 3*(4), 12–19.

Supportive Environments for Health: The Sundsvall Statement. (1991). *Health Promotion International, 6*(4), 297–300.

Susuki, D. (1993). *Time to change.* New South Wales, Australia: Allen & Unwin.

Teilhard de Chardin, P. (1959). *The future of man* (Norman Denny, Trans.). Glasgow: William Collins Sons.

Wheeler, C. E., & Chinn, P. L. (1991). *Peace and power: A handbook of feminist process* (3rd ed.). New York: National League for Nursing.

Wolfe, M. L. (1982). Dimensions of nursing students' attitudes toward the nurse–patient relationship in a patient education setting. *Psychological Reports, 51,* 1165–1166.

World Health Organization. (1981). *Global strategy for Health for All by the Year 2000.* Geneva, Switzerland: Author.

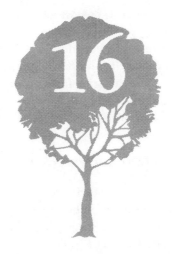

Environmentally Responsible Clinical Practice

Hollie Shaner

ENVIRONMENTAL ISSUES

Environmental issues are continuing to become more and more central to our daily lives. It is vital for nurses to understand the most pressing environmental issues and the consequences to human health resulting from them. *Earth in Balance,* by Vice President Al Gore, introduces the specific issues and likely outcomes. The proceedings from a 1992 conference, "Physicians for Social Responsibility, Human Health, and the Environment," provides a wealth of technical papers addressing the human health consequences identified with a variety of environmental factors, from global warming to loss of biodiversity. The topics covered in this chapter are meant to inform and prepare the practicing nurse as well as to provide specific workplace actions to diminish environmental degradation resulting from clinical practice. In many ways, environmentally responsible clinical practice is nothing more than the transference of one's "at-home" environmentally responsible behaviors to the workplace, be it a hospital, clinic, home, health, or other such setting.

Ozone Depletion

As ozone depletion continues to increase, we can expect an increased incidence of cataracts, melanomas, and other skin cancers in the patient populations we care for. The following quotes, from a paper by McCally and Cassel (1990), suggested what we can expect to find clinically:

Skin Cancer and Melanoma

Reduction in the stratospheric ozone and the resulting increase in ambient ultraviolet radiation would have direct health consequences. The ultraviolet component of sunlight damages skin structure and its immune function. Recent studies have shown that summer sunlight disrupts normal dermal DNA, decreases the effectiveness of antigen presentation, and alters T-cell immune mechanisms. The incidences of both basal and squamous cell carcinoma of the skin are increased by exposure to sunlight. The EPA estimates that for every 1% decrease in atmospheric ozone protection, the incidence of these cancers will increase 4% to 6% in U.S. citizens born before the year 2070. Seasonal ozone depletion over the Antarctic may already be as high as 50%; the "hole" is now the size of a large continent and is increasing.

The incidence of melanoma, an aggressive and commonly fatal cancer associated with sunlight exposure, is increasing worldwide; it is already reaching "epidemic" proportions in light-skinned populations. One author estimated that it has increased 900% in the United States since 1930. Kripke and colleagues recently reviewed the

*potential carcinogenic effects of stratospheric ozone de-
pletion. Their analysis led the EPA to predict a 0.3% to 2%
increase in melanoma incidence among U.S. whites for
each 1% loss of stratospheric ozone. In Australia, television stations already report daily ultraviolet levels and
issue warnings for people to stay indoors when these rise
above a critical level. (p. 469)*

Cataracts

*Epidemiological studies suggest that cataracts are related to
ambient ultraviolet light level. West and coworkers recently
surveyed 838 Chesapeake Bay watermen and found a
strong association between ocular ultraviolet light exposure
and cortical cataract. The EPA ozone depletion scenarios
suggest that many additional cases of cataracts related to
ultraviolet light would be expected in the United States.
Cataracts will be more of a global health problem than
melanoma because cataracts affect all, not just fair-skinned,
populations. In addition, cataract formation and blindness
in animals may also occur, with potential problems for food
production. (p. 470)*

Nursing Action

Become informed about ozone depletion and use that knowledge
to develop prevention programs that focus on sun safety. These
programs might include:

A. Identifying populations at risk, such as farmers, outdoor construction workers, lifeguards, and other professions where the
worker is exposed to the sun for prolonged periods of time in
the course of a regular workday; teaching the use and rationale
for sunscreens, and UV protective eyewear; limiting exposure at
peak times, and so on.

B. Sun Safety Prevention training for children in the public
schools; teaching the use and rationale for sunscreens and UV
protective eye wear; limiting exposure at peak times, and so on.

Global Warming

Increased temperatures will cause changes in weather, sea level, and agriculture, and will affect human health. McCally and Cassel (1990) noted the predicted effects:

> *Global warming will produce increases in the regional temperature gradients that drive wind and storm systems. Weather extremes are very likely to increase. With these extreme episodes of violent weather and weather-related disasters, large new populations of "ecorefugees" from starvation and weather disasters are predicted. The disaster management and international relief communities must plan for these events, which may have already begun. (p. 470)*
>
> *Several features of environmental change make it different from either nuclear war or more common prevention issues in public health, such as smoking or seat belts. First, global warming is unique. For the first time, humans have succeeded in altering the global environment; all human beings are involved. Second, if global warming occurs, the effects on weather, sea levels, and agriculture may result in unimaginable human suffering. We are dealing for the first time with problems of global scale in orders of magnitude more complex and severe than the human species has previously confronted. We must make profound public policy choices in manufacturing, energy, agriculture, and resources, and in our relations to developing countries. Finally, because the pace of environmental change is slow, the threat is not always apparent. (p. 470)*

Nursing Action

A. Identify specific action steps to reduce global warming. Increase utilization of public transportation, energy efficiency, and other actions that will contribute to the minimization of the "greenhouse effect."

B. Learn more about the topic and seek additional ways to help minimize global warming.

C. Support research in this area.

Toxics in the Community

Landrigan (1992) noted that lead poisoning is epidemic among the young in the United States. Lead paint in households continues to be a significant source of exposure to lead in young urban populations. The military has contributed to toxics in the community (O'Toole, 1991).

Nursing Action

A. Identify populations at risk, and target those groups for prevention teaching that includes testing for lead paint in homes and noting proximity to industrial waste sites, military bases, or other potential sources of exposure.

DOCUMENT ENVIRONMENTAL FACTORS OF HEALTH HISTORY

- **WHERE DOES THE PERSON LIVE? DISTANCE TO CLOSEST U.S. MILITARY BASE? PROXIMITY TO INDUSTRIAL AREA?**

- **WHAT DOES THE PERSON DO FOR WORK? WHAT POSSIBLE CHEMICALS IS HE/SHE EXPOSED TO? HOW OLD IS THE BUILDING? HOW IS THE VENTILATION?**

- **WHEN DID THE SYMPTOMS BEGIN? WHEN DO THEY OCCUR? WHERE DO THEY OCCUR?**

ENVIRONMENTAL NURSING
CLINICAL PRACTICE MODEL

• DEVELOP AND DOCUMENT
  ENVIRONMENTAL HISTORY

• CONSIDER ENVIRONMENTAL
  FACTORS RELATIVE TO DIAGNOSIS

• EVALUATE ENVIRONMENTAL
  EFFECTS ON TREATMENT PLAN

B. Take a complete history during a physical assessment. Note home and workplace locations and ascertain their proximity to toxic sites. Identify play areas for children; ensure that children are not allowed to play in abandoned industrial sites.

C. Encourage simple types of testing such as lead testing and radon testing.

Ocean Pollution

Increased pollution, the result of the dumping of multitudes of toxins into our oceans and waterways, is affecting not only the water quality, but the health of the aquatic life that resides within the water. Subsistence fishermen and women are increasingly at risk if they are consuming seafood caught from condemned bodies of water. Immigrants or others not able to read signs posted along contaminated waterways are especially at risk. Research conducted by John Stegeman at Woods Hole Oceanographic

Institution has documented an increasing prevalence of tumors and other diseases among fish. There are correlational links between exposure to specific toxins and the development of the tumors. Ozonoff and Longnecker (1991) have described approaches to assessment of human cancer risk from consumption of food from contaminated water.

Nursing Action

A. Teach seafood safety.

B. Encourage a varied diet.

C. Teach moderation in seafood consumption, especially fatty fish. (It has been documented that the fatty fish tend to bioconcentrate the toxins in their tissues. It has yet to be determined what the effect of excess consumption of contaminated seafood will be. Avoiding bottom feeders may be one strategy to minimize the human exposure to toxins absorbed by the fish.)

Waste Crisis

U.S. hospitals generate over 6,600 tons of waste per day, which is roughly 1%–2% of the total solid waste produced in America daily. Waste has traditionally been disposed of in landfills, and incineration operations, and by dumping. Significant pollution resulting from the illegal dumping of a variety of wastes has caused serious environmental problems. Landfills and incinerators are becoming increasingly difficult to site, for health and aesthetic reasons.

Nursing Action

A. Nurses can understand their role to reduce and recycle wastes in the clinical setting. Solid waste can be source-separated, and a percentage of those materials can be recycled or composted. Regulated medical waste can be minimized by strict adherence to medical waste regulations and by diverting as much nonregulated waste as possible into the solid waste stream. Hazardous wastes, such as mercury, solvents, and batteries, can be minimized in the workplace, and the remaining

- **Minimize use of toxic materials in clinical settings**

  - **Mercury**

  - **toxic cleaning agents**

  - **formaldehyde**

amounts can be properly disposed of. Product substitutions, such as digital thermometers and blood pressure monitoring devices, can be used to decrease the amount of mercury used in clinical settings. Zinc air batteries can be used as substitutes for mercury batteries. Xylene recovery systems can be set up in labs.

B. Nurses can serve on product standards committees and consider the environmental impact of products and their packaging when evaluating them for clinical use. Nurses should seek out and support reuse opportunities for products. Products should be selected for durability rather than disposability.

C. Develop mercury and battery recovery programs in the clinical setting. Clean up the waste stream prior to disposal.

Air Pollution

Florence Nightingale (1992) stated that "the first canon of nursing is clean air." Christiani (1992) noted that "we can expect to

**ISSUES RELATED TO PROCUREMENT OF GOODS
FOR USE IN CARE**

MINIMIZE TOXICITY

- USE DIGITAL THERMOMETERS

- USE DIGITAL/ANAEROID BLOOD PRESSURE MONITORING
  EQUIPMENT

- SEEK PRODUCTS PACKAGED IN BENIGN MATERIALS
- AVOID PVC PACKAGING

- PRACTICE CONSERVATION

**ISSUES RELATED TO PROCUREMENT OF GOODS
FOR USE IN CARE**

- MINIMIZE WASTE

- PURCHASE IN BULK

- SEEK PRODUCTS IN ENVIRONMENTALLY FRIENDLY
  PACKAGING

- ORDER SUPPLIES JUDICIOUSLY

- ONLY ACCEPT SAMPLES YOU WILL USE

ISSUES RELATED TO PROCUREMENT OF GOODS
FOR USE IN CARE

• BUY RECYCLED

* PAPER PRODUCTS

* TRASH CAN LINERS

* TONER CARTRIDGES

* SHARPS CONTAINERS

* TOILET TISSUE & PAPER TOWELS

---

experience an increased incidence of lung cancers, allergies, and asthma in populations in urban areas due to diminished air quality." The effects of poor air quality are continuing to be linked to diminishing respiratory health. Increasingly, in the United States, legislation is being passed that requires public places to be smoke-free.

Nursing Action

A. Advocate smoke-free workplaces.

B. Advocate healthy workplaces, free of "sick building syndrome."

C. Decrease reliance on incineration as a primary disposal option for medical waste management.

D. Support tighter emission control legislation for existing incinerators, and accelerated shutdown plans for polluting incinerators.

ADVOCATE SMOKE-FREE WORKPLACES

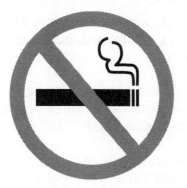

ADVOCATE FOR HEALTHY FACILITIES

FREE OF "SICK BUILDING SYNDROME"

- **PROPER VENTILATION: WINDOWS THAT OPEN AND CLOSE**

- **ENERGY EFFICIENT LIGHTING**

- **WATER-SAVING DEVICES ON ALL FAUCETS, SHOWERS, TOILETS**

ADVOCATE FOR HEALTHY FACILITIES

FREE OF "SICK BUILDING SYNDROME"

- **CAREFUL SELECTION OF CARPETS, CEILING TILES, WALL BOARD AND INTERIOR FURNISHINGS**

- **WELL PLANNED STRUCTURES TO ACCOMMODATE THE CURRENT HEALTH CARE DEVICE TECHNOLOGIES**

- **STRUCTURES WHICH FACILITATE ENVIRONMENTALLY RESPONSIBLE WASTE MANAGEMENT**

Indoor Air Quality

The concept of clean air within buildings has gained much attention recently. Increasing evidence suggesting diminished health effects from poor indoor air quality has been documented. William McClay, an architect from Warren, Vermont, has conducted workshops at various conferences for socially responsible businesses on the importance of fresh, clean air in the workplace. He has specific recommendations and action steps that can be taken by organizations to ensure that the workplace is a "healthy space," free of sick building syndrome. Lost time and decreased productivity from poor indoor air quality have been documented. VOCs and other emissions from carpet, wallcoverings, adhesives, ceiling tiles, paneling, and other construction materials are released into the air. Strategic planning in construction and renovation projects, taking into account the needed time for construction materials to properly off-gas before the area is occupied with personnel, is essential. Selection of materials used in construction, design, and decorating also plays a significant role in the indoor air quality. The implications for health care facilities are enormous, considering that consumers come to a health care facility to get healthy. Health care facilities, foremost among all other facilities, should have clean air and be free of sick building syndrome, because many clients in the health care setting already have compromised health and immune systems.

There are many actions nurses can take to develop their own personal standards for an environmentally responsible clinical practice. Nursing is an art. Each of us can develop our own personal plan to incorporate caring for the environment as well as for humanity. Expanding our scope of knowledge and understanding is a first step. Taking specific actions to minimize the environmental impact of our clinical practice can be a second.

DOCUMENT ENVIRONMENTAL FACTORS OF HEALTH HISTORY

DOES ANYONE IN THE FAMILY SMOKE?

WHAT IS THE FUEL SOURCE USED TO HEAT THEIR HOME?

DOES THE PERSON GET OUTDOORS DAILY?

WHAT IS THE AIR QUALITY LIKE IN THE AREA WHERE THE PERSON RESIDES?

Nursing Action

The following lists suggest specific actions nurses can take to improve the environment.

DAY-TO-DAY, ON-THE-JOB ACTIONS:
THINGS NURSES CAN DO TO SAVE THE EARTH

- ☐ Carpool to work.
- ☐ Recycle newspapers.
- ☐ Use rechargeable batteries.
- ☐ Compost food waste.
- ☐ Recycle magazines.
- ☐ Use a reusable tote sack as a shopping bag.
- ☐ Use popcorn as a packaging material instead of foam peanuts.
- ☐ Wrap gifts in reusable scarves, cloth napkins, a new pair of socks.
- ☐ Turn off water when scrubbing; use only what you need.
- ☐ Recycle glass.
- ☐ Take stairs instead of the elevator.
- ☐ Use cloth napkins.
- ☐ Buy recycled products such as recycled paper, recycled plastic content bags.
- ☐ Substitute less toxic products.
- ☐ Recycle aluminum cans.
- ☐ Share journal subscriptions.
- ☐ Double-side all copies.
- ☐ Route articles instead of copying them.
- ☐ Be an environmental shopper. Precycle—get to know packaging. If you can't recycle or reuse the packaging, consider another product.

☐ Reduce the use of household toxins; read product labels.

☐ Minimize toxic substances in the workplace; phase out the use of mercury-containing products such as thermometers and sphygmomanometers.

☐ Recycle no. 2 HDPE plastic.

☐ Use reusable razors.

☐ Use reusable dishware whenever possible; carry a travel mug in your car.

☐ Buy in bulk.

☐ Become aware of environmental issues and effects; read *State of the World, A Worldwatch Institute Report on Progress Toward A Sustainable Society,* by Lester Brown (1992–1993).

☐ Read *Clean & Green—458 Ways to Clean, Polish, Disinfect, Deodorize, Launder, Remove Stains, Even Wax Your Car without Harming Yourself or the Environment,* by Annie Berthold-Bond (October 1990).

☐ Read *Earth in Balance* by Al Gore.

☐ Keep your car in tune.

☐ Fix leaky faucets.

☐ Use energy-conserving lighting fixtures.

☐ Install water-conserving devices in your home. Request your employer to do so as well.

☐ Teach patients proper disposal for sharps in the home setting.

☐ Only accept from product reps samples that you will use; insist that they take back outdated samples.

ENVIRONMENTALLY RESPONSIBLE ACTIONS FOR NURSES IN CLINICAL SETTINGS (HOSPITALS)

☐ Participate in waste management and chemical right-to-know programs.

☐ Inquire about red-bag waste programs.

☐ Insist on basic recycling in the workplace, for cardboard, paper, cans, glass, magazines, and plastics. Get involved and make it happen.

☐ Request rechargeable batteries for beepers and equipment.

☐ Dispose of chemical waste, mercury spills, and other toxic products in environmentally safe ways. Check with your facility.

☐ Collect unused supplies and divert them to alternate-use settings instead of to trash collection. Nursing schools', veterinarians', and med-tech conservation programs include RACORSE,* and REMEDY.**

☐ Pay attention to product packaging. Request that vendors label products so that they can be recycled.

☐ Share journal subscriptions.

☐ Use reusable dishware whenever possible.

☐ Learn about substitutions for toxic products such as mercury thermometers.

☐ Take stairs instead of elevators.

☐ Practice water conservation when handwashing and doing surgical scrubs.

☐ Carpool to work.

*RACORSE stands for Recycling Allocation and Conservation of Operating Room Supplies and Equipment, an organization designed to assist health care workers to recover and donate unused medical supplies and equipment to the developing world. RACORSE was founded by Lisa Nenonen, of Oakland, California.

**REMEDY is a nonprofit organization founded by Will Rosenblatt, MD, of Yale University, to assist health care organizations to recover and donate unused and discarded medical supplies and equipment to charities in the developing world.

ENVIRONMENTALLY RESPONSIBLE ACTIONS
FOR NURSES IN PUBLIC HEALTH SETTINGS

☐ Use recycled content paper products such as stationery, computer paper, message pads, and business cards. Look for at least a 20% postconsumer content.

☐ Double-side all copies of reports, forms, and printed brochures.

☐ For printed documents, use recycled content paper and soy-based nontoxic inks. Ask your printer to use these products. If they are not available, shop around. More and more printers are becoming aware of environmentally responsible options.

☐ Purchase reusable versus disposable products whenever possible.

☐ Teach your clients to dispose of sharps and contaminated materials properly.

☐ Encourage use of rechargeable batteries.

☐ When on the road, plan efficient routes.

☐ Encourage clients to buy supplies in bulk.

☐ Substitute less toxic materials when possible.

PERSONAL STATEMENT

My personal interest in environmental concerns began when I became a parent. As I watched my infant twins grow, I became more conscious of the environment and the need to preserve its integrity. When my children reached the age of five, we went on vacation to a beach. Trash littering the beach struck a chord deep within me. I had grown up in southeast Florida, visiting beaches frequently. It bothered me that my children had to dodge discarded foam cups, cigarette butts, aluminum cans, pieces of plastic, and glass bottles while playing along the shoreline. The ocean was showing obvious signs of contamination. Most of the "trash" that had washed up on the beach was material that could have been recycled. As I stood at the water's edge, observing my children, I felt something nudging at my ankle. I reached down to examine the object. It was a discarded foam soda can insulator, inscribed with the words "HOLLYWOOD, FLORIDA." I was standing on the beach in York, Maine. The beaches I had played on as a child were in Hollywood, Florida. This event triggered a deep personal commitment within me to do what I could to protect the environment.

Upon returning from vacation, we began to recycle and change our purchasing habits. We eliminated toxic products from our home, and paid more attention to product labels. I was feeling good about my newfound environmental consciousness. I realized that I needed to carry that same sense of responsibility into the workplace. At work, there were few, if any, opportunities to be environmentally responsible. Everything was disposable (paper, packaging, products); nothing was being recycled.

I set out to create opportunities for myself and my colleagues to be environmentally responsible in the workplace. In the process of creating an environmentally responsible clinical practice, I broke new ground. I conducted a research study on operating room waste (MedCycle™ Study), coauthored a book on waste reduction for the health care industry (*An Ounce of Prevention,* published by the American Hospital Association), created a paid position for myself at the Medical Center Hospital of Vermont as the country's first Clinical Waste Reduction Specialist (establishing hospitalwide recycling programs), and started an independent consulting practice, CGH Environmental Strategies, Inc. In the process of all this, I also met my husband, Glenn McRae, the former executive director of The Association of Vermont Recyclers.

I believe that, as health care providers, we must strive to reduce the environmental impact of providing quality health care. That means being careful about the products we choose to provide health care, being responsible about waste disposal, and conserving resources such as water, energy, and other natural resources. I hope that other clinicians will become sensitized to the need to be environmentally responsible in the workplace.

REFERENCES

Berthold-Bond, A. (1990, October). *Clean & green—485 ways to clean, polish, disinfect, deodorize, launder, remove stains, even wax your car without harming yourself or the environment.*

Brown, L. (1992–1993). *State of the world: A Worldwatch Institute report on progress toward a sustainable society.* New York/London: Norton.

Christiani, D. (1992). *Air pollution.* Paper presented at conference of Physicians for Social Responsibility, Cambridge, MA.

Gore, Al. (1992). *Earth in balance.* Boston: Houghton Mifflin.

Landrigan, P. J. (1992). Commentary: Environmental disease—a preventable epidemic. *American Journal of Public Health, 82,* 7.

McCally, M., & Cassel, C. K. (1990). Medical responsibility and global environmental change. *Annals of Internal Medicine, 113*(6), 467–473. Quoted passages reproduced with permission from *Annals of Internal Medicine.*

McClay, W. (1994). *Healthy office interiors: Hands-on information you can use.* Speech before Vermont Business for Social Responsibility, Burlington, VT.

Nightingale, F. (1992). *Notes on nursing: What it is, and what it is not* (p. 9). Philadelphia: Lippincott. (Original work published in 1859.)

O'Toole, T. (1991, February). *Complex cleanup: The environmental legacy of nuclear weapons production.* U.S. Office of Technology Assessment. Washington, DC: Government Printing Office.

Ozonoff, D., & Longnecker, M. P. (1991). Epidemiologic approaches to assessing human cancer risk from consuming aquatic food resources from chemically contaminated water. *Environmental Health Perspectives, 90* 141–146.

Shaner, H., McRae, G., & Bisson, C. L. (1993). *An ounce of prevention.* Chicago: American Hospital Association.

Stegeman, J. (1991). Chemically contaminated aquatic food resources and human cancer risk: Retrospective. *Environmental Health Perspectives, 90,* 149–151.

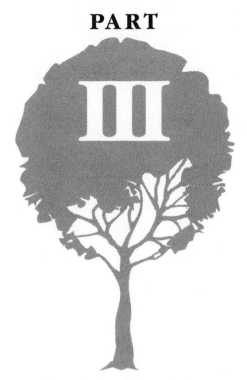

Extending the Domain of Nursing Knowledge through Experiencing

This part presents a variety of experiential perspectives, describing the interplay of experiencing the first nursing conference with an environmental focus. The conference planning committee attempted to create an environment to nurture those participating, honoring them as whole beings interconnected with environment. We invite you to experience the process of a specifically structured nurturing environment with these authors.

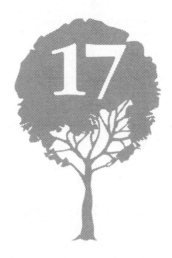

Princesses and Princes from Far and Wide

Patricia L. Munhall

STORYTELLING: A CONFERENCE STORY

I am about to tell you a story. When you were very young, you may have asked your parents, grandparents, or anyone who happened to be there, especially at night, to tell you a story. Often, you would fall asleep during the storytelling. As adults, you probably read stories, often at night, until you fall asleep. (Right now, I am reading a marvelous collection of stories by Martin Amis (1993) called *Visiting Mrs. Nabokov and Other Excursions.*) One thing we need to consider, though it may not always be true, is that we do not fall asleep because the story is boring. Instead, we are lulled to other places and times, and if they are perceived as turning out all right, we relax and sleep follows. In contrast, insomnia comes from perceiving our own lives as they are, in our own time and place. We start thinking about our lives and problems, and wakefulness follows. Television is able to lull people, but that *may* be because of boredom.

This chapter is a bedtime story about a session held at the environmental conference from which this book is derived. I know because I was there. I led the session on storytelling where the topic was the environment.

The Story

Once upon a time, a group of nurses from many different kingdoms came together to discuss caring and the environment. Perhaps not everyone present was an academic nurse, but almost everyone was a nurse and was therefore capable of telling stories, some very long. These very long stories are called dissertations, which give nurses the very worst nightmares.

The nurses, and even those who were not nurses, were all princes and princesses. I know this because they were in Boca Raton, Florida, at the Sheraton Hotel. The skies were clear, the stars were bright, the sand sparkled, and the water was clear, green, and beautiful. I must say, though, that the princes and princesses stayed inside most of the time—a curious phenomenon, considering they were in paradise and were talking about the environment. But they all knew that they "interacted" with the environment, which was indoors as well as outside.

Let me tell you a little bit about Boca Raton. The name brings to mind a song lyric that went something like: "They tore down paradise and built up a parking lot." I exaggerate, but you can do that in stories. A lot of kings and queens who had many treasures lived in Boca Raton, so they built extremely well-guarded, walled-off castles with sentry boxes outside of them. One of the biggest treasures some of the kings and queens had was a swimming pool. This treasure was only a mile or two from the ocean. The Sheraton Hotel also had a pool. And that was where I was for the storytelling session.

Being the head princess (a dream come true), I chose my costume and my story very carefully. I also had Ruth, a friend, help me with some wonderful music to play between stories. I know you are interested in what I wore. I thought it was appropriate to dress like a hippie, because many good ideas about love, peace, and the earth came from the hippies. Besides, this was one of the few times the princes and princesses could dress in jeans at a "professional" conference; this conference had no specific costume expectations. Jeans like mine—one hundred percent natural fibers—are very environmentally *in.* However, I want to tell you something ironic: in Boca Raton, some people wear fur. I hope someone from one of the many castles does not mistake them for live animals.

A Story within a Story

The story I chose to tell is a story within a story. Actually, that is more the case than not, but that is another whole story unto itself. The story I chose was about the North American Indian and the white man. I think it's a good story, and I highly recommend the book of stories and verse where I found it (Wood & Howell, 1974). It tells about terrible things but it's a good story, I thought, about the environment. Like the Amis book, it takes you on excursions. It could have happened in Boca. Indeed, it happened in many kingdoms. With the use of force, the white man took the land away from the Indians. I shut my eyes. I can't even think of all those who were killed outright. This story is a real nightmare, yet we have commercialized it within theme parks and motion pictures—our kingdoms dripping with the blood from massacres on our land, on our earth. They are still happening even as we recycle. Perhaps in my story within a story I wasn't very graphic. We did, though, play some Indian music.

I am truly sorry about the Indians. I know many people are. But many people carry guns and knives. Scattered all over our land are traveling shows of guns and knives. This too is our environment. I wonder: are these "shows" as prevalent where you live as where I live? Last Saturday, I went jogging. I passed the Miami Convention Center in Coconut Grove. I thought to myself, why do they have a monthly gun and knife show here? I was *really* pissed. I felt so powerless. We will come back to feeling powerless again as part of what can help us understand the stories that were told during that night in Boca.

Associations

"That night in Boca": Those words stir a thought of other nights in other kingdoms. "The night they burned Georgia down," and Watts, and parts of "the angels," and Chicago, and the crosses burning on our land, and those ovens . . . nightmare time again.

Our stories during the storytelling session were not about those things. They were not nightmares at all. They were quite lovely stories. Before I tell you about some of those stories, there are two things I must say. First, before this story ends, I will explain why—and even defend why—I think that kings and queens live in Boca. I myself have lived in places called Kings County, where this princess went to nursing school, and Queens County, where this princess practiced nursing.* Second, I must share with you the fact that, as part of preparing for this session, I read *Women Who Run with the Wolves: Myths and Stories of the Wild Woman Archetype* (Estes, 1992). It helped me to get into the spirit of storytelling. For example, not only was I the lead princess, I was the lead *cantadora*. In the role, I kept up an old tradition. At every telling of a story, including this one and the one that night, there is *la invitad*—the guest chair (an empty chair). Sometimes, during the telling, the soul of one or more of the audience comes and sits there, for it has a need to sit there. *La invitad* speaks to the needs of all. As I tell you this story, there is an empty chair in the room. Why do I think my father, who is dead, is sitting there? Is the energy of those whom we think no longer "exist" a part of our environment? Is there an empty chair in the room where you are now? Is someone sitting there?

On that night in the kingdom of Boca, the princes and princesses went along with the head princess, a.k.a. hippie and *cantadora,* and placed the chair in the center of the circle. You know the beginning of the story; I have shared with you a little about the story of the Indian and the white man. Did you know

*Kings County and Queens County are in the City of New York.

that the white man wanted to buy land from the Indians? The Native American Indians, a long time ago, could not even fathom such a concept. The land belonged to itself. It was the earth. No one could own it. No one could own a tree. We certainly have "progressed" when, centuries later, we speak of the shortage of waterfront properties. They are the most valuable pieces, with land, beach, and water. At an environmental conference, we should think about "private property" and "private beaches," and owning trees.

There we were in a circle, with Indian music or what some call, ironically, New Age music, in the background, an empty chair in the center, and the lights low. The kingdom had a fire code against candles, but we managed some. We had a tape recorder to preserve all the stories because many of the princes and princesses (wow, what a slip! I mean princesses and princes, for all the times I have cited the group) were into this German philosopher, Heidegger, and a process called hermeneutics. But that is a story for another night. I just want you to know that we had a tape recorder so that the stories could be "transcribed." In retrospect, I don't know why we didn't go down to the beach, five minutes away and 74° comfortable, and make a campfire. Were we so out of touch with the environment? We do have batteries, so we could even have recorded. When storytelling first started, tape recorders weren't even in existence.

The stories were very interesting. We glimpsed what we associated with stories about the environment. We heard that, for some, a spirit *was* called up to sit in the chair. We heard about children and nature as one, how children really do understand the environment and what it offers. We heard about childhood, vacations, animals, flowers, and farms. If I were to title this story, I would call it "The Garden of Eden." The stories, grouped together, were romantic and idyllic. Even something sad was made good by the environment. Funny how a bite into an apple was the end of that paradise. . . . That apple surfaces again as the beginning of self-determination—and a very big computer company.

I'd like you to read some excerpts from the princesses and princes.

Children Understanding the Environment

One of the princesses told about her little one, a fair miss. One day, while they were walking in the mountains, part of the Garden of Eden, she said, with childlike intuition: "Let's go over that way because that's where life's livings are."

Another princess told of her toddler prince, who loved bedtime stories, especially about animals. Children seem to like animals, sometimes even more than they like people. I should say "other people," because children are people. Sometimes adults treat animals better than they do people. Their tone of voice changes; they become gentle. I could speculate on that in another story, but in this story it does seem that sometimes we separate ourselves from animals as living things. We are living things. We are in the environment, part of the mountains, trees, and animal kingdom. Trouble started here in paradise, I think, when humans began to see themselves as separate from the environment and therefore able to take from the intricate web of life and not give back.

One princess from the Kingdom of Australia remembered that, as a little girl, she went to Cradle Mountain: "It was just magnificent, the colors of Cradle Mountain at the time were white with stars and green with the rain forest."

She went on to say: "My father was a bush man, he actually cut the trees down and I rationalized it by saying that's when they used axes and not front-end loaders."

I wanted to reassure her and say, "As a little girl, how could you know?" But perhaps she did know, in an intuitive way. To a child, with the exception of King George Washington, cutting down trees probably does seem the wrong thing to do. Even King George must have had some inkling, because he lied about it at first, before the virtues of a king came into play. Kings are not supposed to lie—but, let's not get into that.

Another princess at the conference spoke of the mountains in Australia and described sitting on one. She said she felt like she was in a cradle—Mother Earth. The mountain today is known for its bright shades of red—not green; red. Two rhyming words occur to me here: pollution and execution.

My early morning mind-fog wanders before clearing. Right now, I'm recalling an ad for running shoes that boasts, quite unself-consciously: "Hit the Asphalt." Whenever I run, it *is* on asphalt; most runners must run on asphalt. If they run in Central Park, they had best not go north of 100th Street, and, after dark, they probably should not run anywhere in their city kingdom.

A long time ago, children played after dark. Now the law of the land, whether written or unspoken, is to be home before it gets dark. What does this say about our environment and the lack of freedom for our children and ourselves?

About Childhood Vacations

The princesses and princes, that night in Boca, talked also about "vacations," which they associated best with stories about the environment. They recalled staying on farms with cows, chickens, roosters crowing, morning glory flowers, and the smell of rain. Farms are interesting places to think about: farming the land, growing vegetables and fruit, having a garden. In this particular kingdom, the larger one of which I am a part, some farmers are paid *not* to grow crops, because of the effect on the economy, even though people are hungry here and in other places in the world. So much for the spirit of the land. I did fine in economics in college, but the theories seem to leave out the people who are poor or hungry. The homeless are also part of our environment. A fellow princess tells me about capitalism. We all can't be winners, including the environment or the spirit to toil the land. I just think we can do better. That is why the conference was held. That is why this book is being published—to raise our consciousness.

Today, children often have their dream vacation at Disneyland, a world of fantasy. Is that all that is left? No, you say; many families vacation at the beach. Well, last summer, on the Northeast coast, if they did vacation there, children could not go swimming. Do you remember what was being washed up on the shores of those beaches in 1992 and 1993? *Really!* Soon, in some places, there might not be any beaches anyway. Oh, the story is beginning to sound like a nightmare again. Do you know what people say? "It could be worse." Don't worry, that fellow—I can't remember his name—who owns Blockbuster and a whole lot of other things (he's like a vacuum, just sucking up what's in sight) is going to build a huge theme park and recreation area here in Miami. Not far from Miami is the Everglades. One of the princesses at the conference told how her grandfather described the wildlife and vegetation that once existed there. Today, . . . but that too is another story. "Blockbuster"; an interesting word.

The Spirit in the Chair

One prince told a story about a niece who died in an automobile accident at the age of 17. Her name was Sara. The prince did not know Sara well. What he found out about her he learned at her funeral. Sara wrote poetry about the environment and the prince said: "I was so moved by the poetry that was read at her funeral. . . . Though Sara had died, I really knew her in a new way. When you were talking about children's impact on the environment and how they teach us, that also had meaning for me. I realize that, in her own way, she really made an impact as a child on the world."

It seems that Sara's poetry and emphasis on the environment had fostered an environmental consciousness in her school and her town library. I think Sara was sitting in the chair during her uncle's heartfelt remembering of her. Many other individuals sat in that chair during the evening. Memories and stories about grief and losses of those close to the princesses and princes rendered up tales of how in some way animals had helped with recovery from a loss, or stories inscribed on tombstones made the loss easier to bear. From the earth to the earth. So, in that evening, *la invitad* spoke to the needs of all. Sara; three people who were murdered in Tampa; mothers and fathers; children who are now adults—all came from all of our souls and gave of their energy.

The Garden of Eden

No matter what, the stories by the princesses and princes inevitably had happy endings. Nature in its purist form and majesty dominated much of what we might call reality. But this too is reality: when we come together to talk about the environment, we seem to draw on memories of better environmental times—dreamy nights, fresh mornings with dew (yes, dew), fondness for the spirits. Only I, the *cantadora,* added some skepticism. Why was Sara killed in an automobile accident? Why were three people murdered in Tampa?

Boca Raton is like a postmodern Garden of Eden. Kings and queens live there because they feel they may not be murdered. I read somewhere that people today worry less about being mugged or robbed than about being shot. If you live in an armed fortress, the chance that you'll be a victim of crime and violence (unless it's domestic) is much lessened. People can sleep at night, or so they believe. Eleanor and Carolyn, both part of this very volume, do not live behind walls. They live in Boca. Eleanor fondly calls where she lives the "dog patch." I like to think of Eleanor, Carolyn, and myself as kindred spirits. We want a better world, a safer world, a healthy environment. Eleanor developed this whole conference and the storytelling session. She suggested giving back to the earth a piece of what we eat, at each meal, as a symbol of our gratitude for the earth's abundance. However, not everyone has something to give back.

I lived in Boca Raton for one year. I rented what is called a condominium. There was a sentry box outside, with an up-and-down gate; there was high security; and the price to pay for all this was high, both financially and psychologically. I had come from New York City and my being was charged with a sense of impending danger; I was wired for the unexpected terror of city life. (Perhaps I'm getting overdramatic.) In Boca, I experienced withdrawal, so I moved on down to Miami. I think Miami is an absolutely intriguing place. However, here is the environmental paradox. Friends ask: how can I live in Miami? I reply it's a quality-of-life decision. They are quick to point out the violence, the danger. They have not lived in New York City. Some of us like rural living, others urban. But the environmental issues specific to every region must be addressed. A Count I know, from Miami, is moving his family out because of his sense of impending danger. The postmodern Garden of Eden exacts a price.

ALMOST ENDING

My story about the storytelling session is almost ending. Kings and queens in Boca might live happily ever after. Many are there because of their overwhelming feelings of powerlessness against the forces of the night, the immediate environment. Older people can go to the movies at night in that kingdom—usually.

With so many highly credentialed princesses and princes present, you might have thought that our stories about the environment would be more political, perhaps expressing some outrage. Perhaps the souls that sat in the empty chair were gentle and were grateful to see so many come to this consciousness-raising conference. The topics during the day were serious; they had that uniquely academic tone. Perhaps, through the stories, the group expressed wishes for a kinder environment; for fruit, and animals, and exotic vacation lands. Perhaps inherent in the Garden of Eden, as a metaphor for this session, is an unspoken wish for the end of violence, pollution, automobile fatalities, wars, killing of children (one is a child at least 21 years) in wars, toxic anything, disease, homelessness, starvation, and, of course, global warming. In that session, some of us felt we were children again—in that we could believe and imagine. Yet, it seems to me that each of us, in our own way, needs to prioritize our concerns and "Hit the Asphalt" about them. My main concern about the environment is violence in this kingdom. It is part of my situated context. If you live in a place where this is not a problem, perhaps your environmental priority will be different. All of us, royalty or not, should see the intricate environmental web in which we live.

THE STORY ENDING

This tale about a session on a starry, starry night in Boca is ending. The Garden of Eden is what the princesses and princes said they wanted. Their stories tell us something important. Perhaps the past is the plan for the future. Perhaps the price for progress is too costly. Perhaps some of the consequences of progress are illusory.

Progress has made some environmental messes. We are, in some instances, returning to processes of the past to help clean up those messes. For the children of the princesses and princes, we don't want stories to change into nightmares, complete with environmental monsters, robbers, and murderers.

This was a bedtime story about a night in Boca. People gathered to share stories of the beauty of nature, the morning glories, and the ducks. Indian music played, we sang like children, "Happy, Happy Earth Day." Corny as hell, but a bedtime story should be like that—an excursion to a place where all will end well, where the stories have happy endings. That is the way it should be. Or we would never sleep at night.

PERSONAL STATEMENT

Trees, Soil, Water, Air, Rain Forests, and People Care. I suppose these things seem more within the control of humans than human behavior itself. Thus the emphasis on the environment seems to be on nature of the physical sort.

My own worry about the environment has to do with freedom to be with the trees, in the air, or water and on the streets of our towns and cities. The environment can contain carcinogens but somehow what keeps people behind multi-locked doors and gates, and off public transportation, is the *cancer of violence.* The potential exists in every likely or unlikely place. People will remark, "This is not the type of place where a serial killer lurks and then attacks. It took us all by surprise." This is a cancer, a cancer that is dark and growing where we don't know. This is a cancer we fear as much as any other cancer but there is no diagnostic test.

The "cancer of violence" imprisons people. They jump if they hear footsteps, their doorbell, someone on the elevator; they will not go out after dark. What is this, that we call the environment? It includes drug addicts desperate for money, homeless desperate for food, criminals with guns, knives, and clubs. It includes gangs, corrupt officials, and Saturday night specials. The cancer spreads and fear becomes our natural landscape. Something is very, very wrong with our priorities. This, to me is the critical issue in facing environmental problems. What good is clean air, clean water, and talking about the ozone layer, if you can't go out to get a loaf of bread at eight P.M., tonight?!!

REFERENCES

Amis, M. (1993). *Visiting Mrs. Nabokov and other excursions.* New York: Harmony Books.

Estes, C. P. (1992). *Women who run with the wolves: Myths and stories of the wild woman archetype.* New York: Ballantine Books.

Wood, N., & Howell, F. (1974). *Many winters.* New York: Doubleday.

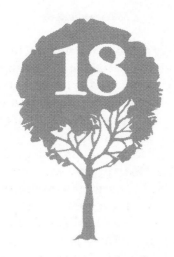

Environmental Messages: Experiencing the Wisdom of the Natural World

Cathy Appleton

LISTENING TO WHAT THE EARTH IS TELLING US

Our relationship with the earth involves something more than pragmatic use, academic understanding, or aesthetic appreciation. A truly human intimacy with the earth and with the entire natural world is needed.

—*Thomas Berry (1988, p. 13)*

The idea of intimacy with the earth and the natural world extends the boundary of the concept of relationship in nursing. The concept of intimacy between the nurse and patient pervades the nursing literature, but intimacy with the earth is novel. Frequently referred to in the nursing literature as an energy field or human bond, the nature of interconnection can now be expanded to include an intimacy with "the entire natural world." Intimacy with the environment provides an interesting and unconventional concept for nurses to use when thinking about what constitutes human presence in nursing.

Berry (1988) states that human presence and intimacy with the natural world involve "listening to what the earth is telling us" (p. 23). Understanding the earth as a unique organism that is self-directed helps us to know we are not alone in determining the course of future events. Berry believes the future depends on the entire earth "in the unity of its organic functioning, on it geological and biological as well as its human members" (p. 23).

This chapter presents dialogue that occurred between the "human members" of the environmental conference represented by this volume. It is about the "geological and biological functioning" of the earth, and the nature of human presence as it was presented in papers, symposia, keynotes, and experiential activities. In an attempt to capture the experience of environmental conference participants, I describe their comments about the natural environment and the conference environment in particular.

NOT A TYPICAL CONFERENCE

Interviewing as many people as possible during the course of the conference, I investigated what the conference was like for each participant. I tape-recorded the descriptions and captured a variety of comments, suggestions, and developing ideas from many interesting and "special" individuals who attended. For example:

> . . . *the openness to accepting different types of approaches and different ways of knowing—that, to me, is special because the people who had the vision made this happen. Secondly, the people who are here presenting are special because they have such diverse perspectives and they have a lot of courage to speak from views that are not widely*

embraced by the rest of nursing per se. Also, the people who are attending I think are special because there is a certain higher level of caring about the environment expressed here. Also, to participate, for instance, in the storytelling, takes a bit of courage to open yourself up to share. It's not a typical thing you see at most nursing scholarship conferences.

"Not a typical conference"; this was a widely held view about the focus of the conference and its participants. "Beyond the traditional conference" referred to the format and focus. With the environment as the central concern, participants described raising consciousness as courageous. Courage was required to participate and to create a forum for new ideas. Many participants expressed a sense that this conference, particularly the focus, was long overdue:

We talk about being progressive, we talk about having a holistic base for our practice, [but] I think there are two areas we do not pay enough attention to; one is the environment and one is spirituality. I think this conference is an awareness or a beginning for us as nurses to hear about the things that we can do that make a difference. It's my reconnection with something as important as the environment.

Reconnecting to the environment and the world we live in describes the perspective that participants overwhelmingly expressed. Realizing the "power of one" to do something for the environment, many participants communicated a sense of power to change the disturbing trends of our times.

Long-established trends affecting the environment appear to be on the decline. For example, the seafood catch per person, growth in the nuclear arsenal, production of chlorofluorocarbons, coal use, and cigarette smoking are decreasing. Driving forces such as population growth and resource utilization continue to threaten the quality of the environment and human life. With the world shifting away from long-established trends that have occurred for decades to more contemporary forces driving environmental change, it's easy to see why Brown referred to the late 20th century as "An Age of Discontinuity" (Brown, 1993, p. 15).

Patterns of human activity that constrain the environment include farming, grazing, fishing, and deforesting activities. Cropland is hardly expanding, and a decent portion of existing agricultural land is losing fertility. Grasslands have been overgrazed, water bodies have endured extensive depletion and pollution, and natural forests continue to recede (Postel, 1994).

What does this mean for the future? According to the *Worldwatch Institute 1993,* emerging protein shortages are on the horizon, leading to scarcity as long as the population continues to grow. If population growth and patterns of human activity continue at present rates, irreversible environmental degradation and continued poverty for much of the world appear inevitable (Brown, 1993, p. 17).

According to Postel (1994), these trends are not new: "Human societies have altered the earth since they began" (p. 3). Unfortunately, as Postel points out, "population and economies grow exponentially, but the natural resources that support them do not" (p. 3).

Three trends that have contributed most directly to the constant strains placed on the natural environment include: (1) the doubling of the world population, (2) the quintupling of the global economic output, and (3) the widening gap in the distribution of income. Of these three trends, Postel (1994) believes the "chasm of inequity" is a major cause of environmental decline. Surprised and amazed participants heard about the outcome and effects of these trends from international presenters, "people from Australia, from Iceland, from Africa, from Canada," who gave them "a whole new perspective" by:

> *. . . explaining to us why we need to care for the ozone, the global warming and the changing of environmental conditions. People are having to walk for water and wood. We talk about the ozone, that people can actually be dying, and really dying because of what's happening in the environment as the result of those changes in our everyday world.*

Participants interviewed stated that caring for the environment was not only essential to a humanistic practice of nursing, but could influence some of the more contemporary environmental trends we experience today.

A survey of 42 global indicators compiled for the *Worldwatch Institute 1993* essentially showed that policy makers face four fundamental challenges: (1) the difficulty of expanding the production of basic foodstuffs, such as grain, seafood, and livestock products, as fast as the growth of the population; (2) the inability of the global economy to expand as easily as it once did; (3) the arrival of a basic restructuring of the world energy economy; and (4) the continuing rapid population growth that shows signs of undermining living standards (Brown, 1993, pp. 15–16).

These trends provide challenges that require a new perspective about human–environment well-being. At a human level, well-being has always been viewed by nurses in terms of effective cultivation and use of resources for the aim of promoting human growth and development. However, when considering the environment and trends of human patterns of activity, an expanded understanding of what constitutes growth and well-being is required. Population expansion and depletion of environmental resources—both patterns of human activity—have diminished well-being for the environment and its inhabitants.

Historically, nurses have identified the significance of the environment for human health and healing. Nightingale (1969/1859), for example, emphasized the role of the environment in her model of nursing. Rogers (1970, 1987) specifically explicated the human–environment relationship as energy fields in her theory of Unitary Human Being.

More recently, Schuster (1990) identified the need to explore the interrelationship of environment, nursing, and caring. Challenging nurses to extend "the apparent anthropocentric emphasis of current human care and caring theory," Schuster cautioned us about particularizing caring to humankind (p. 25).

Notwithstanding these scholars and others, participants at this conference talked about the need for increasing attention to the environment as a focus, even a "domain" of the nurse's caring that has yet to claim a central position to a practice of nursing as healing.

MAKING CONSCIOUSNESS CONSCIOUS

*Most often, we think of the natural world as an economic re-
source, or as a place of recreation after a wearisome period
of work, or as something of passing interest for its beauty on
an autumn day when the radiant colors of the oak and
maple leaves give us a moment of joy. All these attitudes
are quite legitimate, yet in them all there is what might be
called a certain trivializing attitude. If we were truly moved
by the beauty of the world about us, we would honor the
earth in a profound way. We would understand immediately and turn away with a certain horror from all those activities that violate the integrity of the planet.*

—Thomas Berry (1988, p. 10)

"Being moved profoundly" about what was said about the environment and the experience of the environmental conference
jumps off the pages of transcripts from participants' interviews.
For example, participants spoke of feeling cared for while engaging in storytelling, yoga, and massage—activities designed for self-
exploration, reconnection, and rejuvenation. They described the
organization of the conference as "demonstrating caring both personally and within the collective [as a whole]."

In addition to being profoundly moved, participants described
their sense of a sacred experience:

*. . . after Jean Watson's presentation yesterday, the silence in
that room was so profound, people didn't even move in their
seats. People didn't look at their watch, or squirm, nobody
got uncomfortable. I thought that was remarkable. My sense
was that she altered consciousness and people were in a
trance. I mean that in the most positive sense, an inter-
reflective state from having had a very sacred experience.*

Naess's (1988) concept of an *ecological self,* the richer consti-
tutive relations of the self with the larger community of the natural world (p. 20), captures the consciousness made conscious in

Watson's (1992) keynote address, perhaps contributing to what one participant called a sense of the sacred.

Naess (1988) made six points in describing an ecological approach to Being-in-the-world:

1. We underestimate ourselves because we tend to confuse *self* with the narrow *ego.*

2. Human nature is such that, with sufficient all-sided maturity, we cannot avoid "identifying" ourselves with all living beings.

3. Traditionally, the *maturity of the self* develops through three stages—from ego to social self and then to metaphysical self.

4. Increased self-realization implies broadening and deepening the self.

5. Because of the process of identification, self-realization is hindered if the self-realization of others, with whom we identify, is hindered. Love of ourself will labor to overcome this obstacle by assisting in the self-realization of others, according to the formula "Live and let live." All that can be achieved by altruism—the dutiful, moral consideration of others—can be achieved—and much more—through widening and deepening ourself. Following Immanuel Kant's critique, we then act beautifully but neither morally nor immorally.

6. The challenge of today is to save the planet from further devastation that would violate the enlightened self-interest of both humans and nonhumans, and would decrease the potential of joyful existence for all. (pp. 19–21)

"That with which the person identifies" is what Naess (1988, p. 22) referred to as the ecological self. Like Berry (1988), Naess broadened the concept of self-in-relation. Based in a theoretical perspective about the human capacity of identification, Naess's *metaphysical self* and Berry's concept of *intimacy with the natural world* offer an interesting awareness about living nonviolently, a practice that does not moralize but just cultivates the capacity to act beautifully.

Nursing, as a practice, stands to be enriched by Naess's (1988) notion of the ecological self and Berry's (1988) concept of intimacy with the natural world, two distinct phenomena existent when nurses practice nursing as an art (Appleton, 1991). Consistent with the findings of what constitutes the art of nursing is the idea of an ecological self and intimacy with the natural world, both described in Abendroth's (1986) nine principles of a feminist aesthetic (Appleton, 1991).

For example, Abendroth's first and second aesthetic principles include the idea that matriarchal art influences reality based on a perspective of the whole. This perspective unifies the individual, society, and nature into a wonderful harmony, and recognizes the diversity in the unity that exists as an enduring implicit universal structure and explicates this structure into the modern consciousness (p. 84–88).

Naess's notion that living beautifully stems from an ecological approach to Being-in-the-world is consistent with Abendroth's feminist aesthetic principles and the belief that a paradigm of practice exists for designing nursing as art, a practice of nursing that is beautiful and encompasses the perspective of an ecological selves? (Appleton, 1991, 1994).

THE ENVIRONMENT THAT LIVES IN YOUR SPIRIT

. . . we must find and develop therapies which heal our relations with the widest community, that of all living beings.

—Arne Naess (1988, p. 29)

Venolia (1988) recommended, "As you explore your inner landscape and its outward projections, you will be healing both yourself and your world. That sense of integration—of the power to perceive, nurture, and actualize—can bring increasing harmony and wholeness" (p. 37).

What does the practice of nursing say about our inner landscape and its outward projection? About how we relate to the natural world and its inhabitants? Does the concept of health, being, and caring expand our consciousness of intimacy with the natural world? Which parts of these concepts receive the most attention?

Which parts do we neglect? Does anything we do in nursing encourage us to grow and express our ecological self?

Participants described being impressed with the possibilities of creating healing environments:

> *I was very impressed with Charlie's (Beauchamp, 1993) presentation. He wanted to talk about creating a nursing environment in which people could be, and he really lived that presentation as he was with us. He talked about what was happening in hospices, the work he was doing. I was really moved because when nurses were in charge of the environment, they were able to make the difference in what went on; the patients got better. And when you talk about patients getting better that are hospice patients, I think that's a significant statement to make.*

Not only is this statement significant, but it reflects the responsibility nurses have to "design" nursing so that well-being means vitality in terms of the whole (Appleton, 1994). Healthy environments are vital, nurturing, and self-sustaining. Good health means participating in "the dynamic web of life," in deriving nourishment from the natural world, and, in turn, contributing creativity, labor, vision, and love (Venolia, 1988, p. 7).

In summary, understanding intimacy as the bridge between knower and known describes the environmental message participants received from this conference. Raising awareness that intimacy is not restricted to human relationships, but extends from humans to the natural world, and from the natural world to humans, reflects the wisdom of the environment.

PERSONAL STATEMENT

I've possessed an interest in and awe for the natural world as long as I can remember. As a youngster, I always lived close to waterways (rivers and oceans), in a small town that consisted of farmland with dairy farms in the outlying areas. This surrounding provided the context from which an appreciation of the natural world developed.

Learning about and how to live with the environment began during my formative years and was maintained throughout my academic experience. Having multiple academic interests, I enrolled in courses that helped me recognize the practices (my own and those of others) that contribute to the demise of the natural world. In addition, academics provided me the opportunity to cultivate a worldview that encompasses many of the ideas described in this chapter.

In my lifetime, both personal and professional experiences have contributed to my interest in and ongoing development of ideas and knowledge about the nature of relationships within the context of the natural world and beyond. Living a commitment to honor the natural environment has taken shape for me in my daily activities, in the professional memberships that I hold, and in conferences and workshops that I attend. With each of these endeavors, I become increasingly hopeful and concerned about the human–environment evolution.

REFERENCES

Abendroth, H. (1986). Nine principles of a matriarchal aesthetic. In G. Ecker (Ed.), H. Anderson (Trans.), *Feminist aesthetics* (pp. 81-94). Boston: Beacon Press. (Original work published 1985.)

Appleton, C. (1991). The gift of self: The meaning of the art of nursing. *Dissertation Abstracts International, 52,* 12B. (University Microfilms No. 92-15, 314.)

Appleton, C. (1994). The gift of self: A paradigm for originating nursing. In P. L. Chinn & J. Watson (Eds.), *Art and aesthetics in nursing* (pp. 91-114). New York: National League for Nursing.

Beauchamp, C. (1993). *Nursing: Toward a heavenly harmonization with and while on earth.* Presentation conference on expressions of caring in nursing: Exploring our environmental connections. See Chapter 14, this volume.

Berry, T. (1988). *The dream of the earth.* San Francisco: Sierra Club Books.

Brown, L. (1993). Overview: An age of discontinuity. In L. Starke (Ed.), *Vital signs 1993: The trends that are shaping our future* (pp. 15-22). New York: Norton/Worldwatch Books.

Naess, A. (1988). Self-Realization: An ecological approach to being in the world. In J. Seed, J. Macy, P. Fleming, & A. Naess (Eds.), *Thinking like a mountain: Toward a council of all beings* (pp. 19-30). Philadelphia: New Society Publishers.

Nightingale, F. (1969). *Notes on nursing: What it is, and what it is not.* New York: Dover. (Original work published in 1859.)

Postel, S. (1994). Carrying capacity: Earth's bottom line. In L. Starke (Ed.), *State of the world: A Worldwatch Institute report on progress toward a sustainable society* (pp. 3-21). New York: Norton/Worldwatch Books.

Rogers, M. E. (1970). *An introduction to the theoretical basis of nursing.* Philadelphia: Davis.

Rogers, M. E. (1987). Nursing: A science of unitary human beings. In R. R. Parse (Ed.), *Nursing science: Major paradigms, theories, and critiques* (pp. 139-146). Philadelphia: Saunders.

Schuster, E. (1990). Earth caring. *Advances in Nursing Science, 13*(1), 25-30.

Venolia, C. (1988). *Healing environments.* Berkeley, CA: Celestial Arts.

Watson, J. (1993). *A frog, a rock, a ritual: Myth, mystery, and metaphors for an ecocaring cosmology in a universe that is turning over.* Keynote address, conference on Expressions of Caring in Nursing: Exploring Our Environmental Connections. See Chapter 2 of this volume.

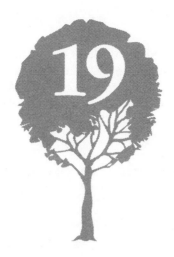

Face Painting as Metaphor

Charlotte D. Barry

Exploration was the theme of this conference, and flights of fancy were encouraged. Participants were invited to build on basic environmental nursing notions like controlling effluvia (Nightingale, 1969/1859), and to recreate the meaning of environment for nursing. What better way to dream and envision new ways of being than to be in a milieu where different ways of thinking were encouraged and different ways of participating were respected and celebrated? Face painting was a metaphor for letting go of the routine and envisioning a prism of environmental connections for nursing.

The purpose of this paper is to publicly 'fess up to designing a corner of whimsy at the environmental conference. Rabbits and angels "took tea and cookies," and participants and presenters sat among stars and streamers to have their faces painted. The purpose of the corner was to create a comfortable surrounding where persons connected through touch and where the usual serious business of nursing and learning were set topsy-turvy. In this corner, scholars were invited to be open to the experience of playful laying on of hands, to let their creativity be energized, and to dream of possibilities for caring for themselves, the environment, and nursing.

PERSPECTIVES ON ENVIRONMENT, ART, TOUCH, AND FUN

My perspective of the interrelatedness of all living matter has been informed by many sources, known and unknown. I offer some of the published works that I've enjoyed about the environment, art, touch, and fun that helped shape my notion that face painting would be right for this environmental conference.

Environment

The environment has been an important concept in modern nursing. As articulated by Nightingale (1969/1859), it is the immediate environment surrounding the patient—air, odors, light, noise, and warmth. Nightingale also pointed up the social settings that contribute to health and illness. Other nursing scholars, most notably Lillian Wald, have taken this broader view. Wald, after witnessing firsthand the hardships of poverty and disenfranchisement, created the Henry Street Settlement House as a center of caring and concern for the poor of lower Manhattan (Kelly, 1985).

More than 100 years later, nursing scholars have prompted a thoughtful refocus on the notion of environment (Chopoorian, 1986; Kleffel, 1991; Schuster, 1990). Chopoorian called for nurses to expand the notion of environment to include not only the immediate and mundane context of our patients' lives but to think of the relationships between health and the social issues that ". . . influence human beings and hence create conditions for health and illness . . ." (p. 53). Calling for a paradigm shift, Kleffel urged nurses to move the concept of environment "upstream" and examine all that we have failed to see: vast social, political, economic, and cultural injustices and inequities that keep many of our patients and ourselves from enjoying "mainstream" life and health.

Schuster's reflections on earth caring inspire another look at the environment. Asserting that most published nursing literature on caring is focused on human-to-human caring, Schuster asks the reader to consider a broader view of caring that includes nonhuman species and the physical world. Acknowledgment of the interrelatedness of all living things energizes caring from this broader perspective into a wider circle.

Touch

The laying on of hands is one of the oldest therapies applied to the sick, as illuminated in the Christian parables of healing. Likewise, for centuries, Chinese medicine has advocated using hands to apply pressure and seek out diseased spots. I think one of the fullest descriptions of touch is offered by Meister Eckhart in describing spiritual humility: ". . . being in touch with the earth, in touch with one's own earthiness" (cited in Fox, 1973, p. 59). Barry (1993) offered that touch connects humans to each other, grounding the nurse to the nursed in nursing's value of humility.

Rogers (1971) gave us a different lens with which to view touch and the environment. This perspective, based in physical science, posits human beings and the environment as energy fields in constant interaction with each other, moving toward greater complexity, changing both human beings and environment. The concept of environment in Rogerian science has inspired nursing scholars to examine energy with particular attention to touch.

Krieger (1979) studied the phenomenon of touch and developed a model of nursing practice focused on energy patterns both within and outside the patient. "Therapeutic Touch" (Krieger, 1979) seemed to heal human beings, as reflected in measurable physiologic changes. This very specific method of touch is conducted by many nurse healers who confirm therapeutic changes in themselves as well as in their patients.

Art

Tomas (1968; cited in Boykin, Parker, & Schoenhofer, in press) wrote: "To create is to originate." Creativity stems from many unseen and unknown wells, and crystallizes into an unpredicted apprehension of the spirit. The art reflects the artist as well as the viewer, creating anew the experience of the genesis of imagination. The audience becomes participants (Boykin et al., in press).

"All art unites, it is a means of communication and moves humanity toward well-being" (Tolstoy, 1930, cited in Boykin et al., in press). The nurse, as artist, seeks aesthetic pathways that unite her or him to patients and colleagues.

> *The nurse artist has heightened awareness of relationships, circumstances and environments. She values, looks for and creates connections of her art and her nursing. She is truly present with her patients and brings forth interactions of art and nursing for the possibilities of healing. (Parker, 1992, pp. 34–35)*

Fun

Norman Cousins laughed himself well, and asserted humor as a healing essence. *The Reader's Digest,* the most widely read magazine in the United States, has promoted laughter as the best medicine for many years. This feature pokes fun at serious problems and, often, at serious medical persons.

Adams (1993), a physician and clown, joyfully tells us that "health is based on happiness from hugging and clowning around to finding joy in family, friends, satisfaction in work, and ecstacy in nature and the arts" (p. 1). This physician has practiced medicine for the past 20 years, building on humor, joy, and love to focus on nurturing, healing relationships. He currently publishes a newsletter called "Achoo," which promotes this philosophy through news from the "Gesundheit Institute." The Institute is in the process of building a model medical community and "silly hospital" devoted to humor and healing.

The above thumbnail sketch of sources that informed me about the possibilities of face painting provides a view of the nature of the four concepts: (1) environment, (2) touch, (3) art, and (4) fun. More importantly, the literature review helps illuminate the relationships between and among the concepts. The impact of the environment on all living things points up the need to thoughtfully create nurturing surroundings where each living thing has the chance to grow, flourish, and enhance the growing and flourishing of each other living thing.

THE FACE PAINTING EXPERIENCE

Jane Adams, a nurse artist, and I arranged our individual work stations at our decorated and festooned table. We sat sideways to the table and each of us had another chair ready for our cocreators of this experience. We displayed samples of our designs and asked each person to select. Some would select, some would ask each of us to select, and some asked us to design something new.

Half moons, stars, rainbows, lightning bolts, suns, globes, flowers, clouds, trees, and birds were created on cheeks, necks, hands, arms, and legs. The designs were done with water-based nontoxic crayons, usually in vibrant colors. Often, the designs were sprinkled with glitter which not only gave a sparkling radiance to the designs, but could also be used to cover up any unsightly misplaced blobs of color.

Once initiated, the face painting took on a life of its own. Jane and I began to experience a heightened awareness of our presence and touch with our cocreators. The cocreator, once introduced and seated, settled into what seemed to be a state of mutuality and trust with us. As Jane and I concentrated on the designs and held the person's face, hand, or leg, the person would begin to share the experience of this activity.

This artistic activity unfolded and laid open to us possibilities not dreamed of. Our playful laying on of hands seemed to be having a remarkable effect, and we began to write down our cocreators' responses to face painting.

RESPONSES TO THE EXPERIENCE

It means being reanointed to feel and be with the environment. A tree is something to cherish, it keeps us going, gives shelter, fuel, fruits, shade to sit under in the hot sun, to reflect on one's own being, to reflect on what God put you on earth to do.

It feels like going back to Indian roots.

I love being attended to.

*I thought the sense of touch, I felt the touch on my face—the
pressure so close to my eyes—I felt trust. It was fun afterward having it on my face—looking in the mirror after I
took a pee. Drawing on my face was pleasant and interesting, like a massage.*

*It feels unbalanced, I need the other side to be touched.
Touching my head and face feels so good.*

*I avoided coming; I felt it was risky. Then I felt the child
should be free and I knew you would know what to put on
my face.*

*I needed to be touched, to be held, to be cared for, I just fin-
ished my presentation.*

*The experience helped people open up to me, they talked to
me a lot. In choosing the motif, they selected a symbol that
expressed who they were or what they were feeling. I sensed
the fragility of each person, I had to be careful about what
I was doing, working so close to the eyes. If the person asked
me to choose, I had to decide what was just right for that
person. (Jane Adams, nurse artist)*

The responses are shared for the reader's reflections. No attempt has been made to interpret the data. No attempt has been
made to draw conclusions or offer recommendations.

OTHER LEADINGS

This chapter describes an experience of caring that had an immediate impact on the environment. Jane and I thoughtfully and

carefully established a corner for comfort and fun; a special place to experience caring. The table was whimsically and artistically decorated to celebrate our coming together. The offer of earth-friendly face designs announced a different type of caring for a different sort of gathering. We hoped face painting would contribute to the artistic visionary work of the conference.

We intentionally created an environment where possibilities were dreamed of. We intentionally offered presence and touch as communion. We intentionally expressed caring in nursing as a thoughtful art. And we, as nurse artists, were blessed with creating and experiencing the vibrant, shimmering strands of connections between nursing and the environment.

PERSONAL STATEMENT

My awakening to the interrelatedness of living things came in the early 1960s. My friend and I stayed awake for hours in a candle-lit room listening to Peter, Paul, and Mary plaintively inquire: "Where have all the flowers gone?" The words to this folk song inspired an understanding of the circular motion of things. A second awakening came to me in 1970, the first celebration of Earth Day. My husband and I joined many other New Yorkers walking on 14th Street in Manhattan, to demonstrate our budding awareness of Mother Earth as a sacred, fragile environment. Attending this celebration was considered slightly subversive. Rachel Carson was still being blasted at this point as being fanatical, while oil blobs floated in and polluted the beautiful California coastline.

My third and more startling awakening came as the destruction and waste moved into my neighborhood and permanently into my consciousness. Mountains made of garbage were being built in Florida. The pristine waters off the coast, particularly in the Keys, were not as clear as they had been. The large sugar cane growers and farmers were pouring contaminants into our drinking water source, the ozone layer was being depleted, reports were coming in about huge slicks of garbage floating in the middle of the ocean, and the primordial rain forests in Central America were being destroyed to raise cattle for McDonald's hamburgers.

I sustain myself by learning more and trying to do my part. I started a recycling program for paper and aluminum at my daughter's grade school. My children inspire me to do more. My daughter boycotts fast-food eateries, and my son calculates commonly consumed items to determine packaging waste. We are all members of a global community, and when that famous tiny butterfly flaps its wings in South America, we feel the breeze here.

REFERENCES

Adams, P. (1993). *Gesundheit.* Rochester, VT: Healing Arts Press.

Barry, C. D. (1993). *The values lived in the day-to-day practice of nursing.* Unpublished master's thesis. Florida Atlantic University, Boca Raton.

Boykin, A., Parker, M. E., & Schoenhofer, S. O. (in press). Aesthetic knowing grounded in an explicit conception of nursing. *Nursing Science Quarterly.*

Chopoorian, T. (1986). Reconceptualizing the environment. In P. Moccia (Ed.), *New approaches to theory development* (pp. 39-54). New York: National League for Nursing.

Fox, M. (1973). *Original blessing.* Santa Fe, NM: Bear and Company.

Kelly, L. (1985). *Dimensions of professional nursing.* New York: Macmillan.

Kleffel, D. (1991). Rethinking the environment as a domain of nursing knowledge. *Advances in Nursing Science, 14*(1), 40-51.

Krieger, D. (1979). *The therapeutic touch.* Englewood Cliffs, NJ: Prentice-Hall.

Nightingale, F. (1969). *Notes on nursing: What it is, and what it is not.* New York: Dover. (Original work published in 1859.)

Parker, M. (1992). Exploring the aesthetic meaning of presence in nursing practice. In D. Gaut (Ed.), *The presence of caring in nursing* (pp. 25-37). New York: National League for Nursing.

Rogers, M. (1971). *Theoretical basis of nursing.* Philadelphia: Davis.

Schuster, E. (1990). Earth caring. *Advances in Nursing Science, 13*(1), 25-30.

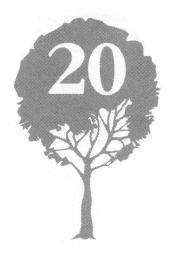

Environmental Connections
and Reawakened Spirit

Margaret A. Burkhardt

INTRODUCTION

This paper suggests that renewal of spirit is at the heart of living our interconnectedness with all of life. My research with Appalachian women is the basis for a model that views spirituality as a unifying force that is, at its heart, relational. Caring connections with self, others, nature, and God or Ultimate Other shape the context within which, and through which, one's spirituality is experienced. In this model, connecting with Ultimate Other includes being with others and being in nature, as well as participation in personal prayer, meditation, ritual, or church-related activities. A sense of connectedness to the earth and of deriving strength from nature is a strong element in this understanding of spirituality. Appreciating, respecting, and caring for nature are discussed as ways of expressing and experiencing spirituality. Connectedness with others incorporates the living-out of relationships, which may be loving or painful, difficult or supportive. These relationships—with family, friends, and others—involve receiving as well as giving, and a sense of the flow of life from one generation to another. A unity in the process of interconnectedness embraces all of life and is made whole by living it. It is within the self that spirituality is experienced and expressed. Relationship with self, a core manifestation of spirituality, encompasses one's being (the essence of who one is), one's knowing (both content and process), and one's doing (the actions of living). Reawakening spirit is essential to the healing of ourselves and of our world. Ways in which nurture of the spirit can be facilitated in ourselves and with others are discussed.

The awareness that there are no real separations—rather, that all things are connected—is a manifestation of spirit. Spirituality opens us to the awareness of our connectedness with all in our environment. Spirit and spirituality are a part of us, having been within our lives and world throughout time. Green (1986) suggested that spirituality is the information nexus binding things, people, and the world together, informing each of its nature and context. Etymologically, the words *spirit* and *spirituality* are derived from the Latin word for breath, which might suggest that spirituality is as fundamental to life as the act of breathing (Clifford & Gruca, 1987). This is reflected in one of the Judeo-Christian creation accounts, which notes that after God fashioned "Adam" from the soil (Adam means "of the soil"), the breath of life was breathed into Adam's nostrils (Gen 2:7). It can also be seen in references to Wisdom as a breath of the power of God (Wis 7:25), which was with God through the process of creation and is at play everywhere in God's world (Prov 8:22–31).

Somehow, however, we humans, at least those of us in Western, industrialized societies and cultures, seem to have fallen asleep and become anesthetized to the reality of spirit in all of life. In our busy lives, which keep us inside homes and other buildings, in which we ride in cars rather than walk, buy food grown by others, and have learned to put great value in science and technology, we can easily be distanced from the earth. In the midst of these distractions, we have come to believe that perhaps we are the only beings on the earth with souls, spirits, or real intelligence, and that this gives us the right, and obligation, to "subdue" the earth, to do with it what we will. For these and other reasons, we seem to have lost sight of the truth expressed by Chief Seattle (Jeffers, 1991): we do not weave the web of life, we are but a strand in the web.

We are beginning to recognize anew that what happens to one of the strands in the web affects the whole, and what we do to the web, we do to ourselves. We have experienced this in things like the worldwide effects of major volcanic eruptions, and we are coming to appreciate that the destruction of major ecosystems such as rain forests affects the environment of all the earth. The indigenous peoples of this continent, whom we call Native Americans, teach us that spirit is in all of life, and thus we are sisters and brothers with rocks, trees, plants, birds, water creatures, all four-legged as well as two-legged beings. We must learn to live this interconnectedness if we are to truly bring healing to ourselves and our world.

INTERCONNECTEDNESS: A RENEWAL OF SPIRIT

This chapter suggests that renewal of spirit is at the heart of living our interconnectedness with all of life. An underlying assumption is that the unitary nature of the human person is manifest in physical, mental, emotional, and spiritual ways. Many authors have described spirit as the unifying force and animating principle of the person (Burkhardt, 1989). It has been suggested that spirituality is an important factor in health and healing (Burkhardt & Nagai-Jacobson, 1994; Carson, 1989; Mickley, Soeken, & Belcher, 1992; Nagai-Jacobson & Burkhardt, 1989; Siegel, 1986; Stiles, 1990; Stuart, Deckro, & Mandle, 1989). However, by its very nature, spirit remains elusive and difficult to quantify or describe. The whole idea of addressing spirit or spirituality tends to scare many people, especially those of us in health care professions. Perhaps we feel that if we do not have a degree in theology, or know about religious traditions, or at least pray on a regular basis, we cannot understand and are not prepared to deal with spiritual issues.

The lack of clarity related to understandings of spirituality presented in the nursing literature led to my research in this area. Although the literature speaks of spirituality in terms such as personal
transcendence, meaning and purpose in life, life-affirming relationships, and relationship with God or Universal Force, research
has often focused on one's relationship with God and on religious
practices, primarily from a Judeo-Christian perspective (Burkhardt,
1989). Measurements of spirituality frequently have included
prayer, bible reading, requests for pastoral care visits, and other religious beliefs and practices. This would suggest that spirituality is
only present or active if a person believes in a God, which contra-
dicts the presumption that spirit is an essential manifestation of a
human person.

Much of my research related to spirituality has focused on
women, because women's experiences have been poorly documented; in the age of "*his*tory," "*her*story" has not been told. The
model of spirituality that I present here flows primarily from a
grounded theory study that explored understandings of spirituality among women in Appalachia (Burkhardt, 1993). I acknowledge
that a qualitative investigation with 12 women is not sufficient for
generalization of the findings. However, the themes identified here
are consistent with reports of other studies focused on spirituality
found in the literature (Anderson & Hopkins, 1991; Barker, 1989;
Burkhardt, 1993), which lends support to this evolving model.

The women who participated in this study have much to teach
us. Because I would like you to hear their stories, I will use their
words as much as possible. First, let me introduce you to the participants, identified using coded initials, and briefly describe the
study. This study included women who had lived in Appalachia all
of their lives, and women who had adopted the region as their home.
Participants have lived in both rural and urban areas. Demograph-
ics for the women are summarized in Tables 20–1 and 20–2.

Participants for this study were recruited through primary health
care centers where I had worked and through personal contacts
within the community. In order to participate, women had to be 18
years or older, living in Appalachia, not hospitalized, and willing to
be interviewed. I contacted the participants initially by phone to
explain the study, and collected written informed consent at the

Table 20–1   Demographic Data (N = 12)

Age Range in Years		Years of Residence in Appalachia		
30–39	3	Lifelong	30–50	6
40–49	6		50–80	2
50–80	3	Nonlifelong	15–32	4

Marital Status		Number of Children	
Married	6	None	1
Single	1	1–2	7
Divorced	2	3–4	4
Widowed	3		

Educational Experience

Did not complete high school	2
High school+other training	4
Completed college+other courses	5
Completed Master's degree	1

Occupations

Hairdresser	Research Field Coordinator/Nurse
Medical Receptionist	Bank Loan Officer
Health Educator	Personnel Technician
Social Worker (retired)	Perinatal Coordinator
Housewife/Mother (retired) (2)	Health Care (between jobs)
Adolescent Pregnancy Specialist	

face-to-face interview. All interviews were audio tape-recorded and lasted for about one hour. The opening question, "What do you understand by the term *spirituality?*" was the same for each participant. Subsequent questioning to gain depth and clarity was guided by the participant's response. Prior to the analysis, each transcript was reviewed with the participant for clarification and validation of accuracy. Data were analyzed utilizing the constant comparative processes described by Glaser and Strauss (1967) and Lincoln and Guba (1985). The synthesized description of spirituality was reviewed with each participant for accuracy in reflecting her understanding of spirituality, and was validated by each.

Interconnectedness was clearly a major element of spirituality for the women, as reflected in the synthesized description of spirituality. I will first present the description of spirituality that was

Table 20–2 Demographic Data (N = 12)

Self-Described Ethnic Background and Race

Black	Norwegian/Caucasian
Scotch-Irish/Caucasian	Irish/American Indian/White
Pennsylvania Dutch/White	American Indian/Dutch/White
German-Dutch/White	African American
Scotch-Irish/Caucasian	Liberal/S. California/White
Polish/Jewish/White	Eastern European (Polish/ Yugoslavian/German/ Croatian)/Caucasian

Religious Affiliation*		Religious Activities Practiced
Methodist	1	Church/Sunday School
Christian	2	Choir/Church circles
Baptist	2	Prayer
Jewish	1	Rituals, e.g. Seder, chanting
Unitarian/Quaker	1	
None	5	

Spiritual Discipline Practiced

Meditation/Visualization	Praying
Fasting	Reading
Moments of silence	Walking
Group rituals	

*Six of those noting a particular religious affiliation claimed to be active members, attending church 1-3 times per week or services 3-4 times per year.

affirmed by the participants, and will then flesh out how it speaks to connectedness, particularly with nature and environment. In the understanding of these women, spirituality is:

> *The unifying force that shapes and gives meaning to the pattern of one's self becoming. This force is expressed in one's being, in one's knowing, and in one's doing, and is experienced within the context of caring connections with self, others, nature, and God or Higher Power.*

Spirituality involves that which gives meaning within one's life journey. The self is central, for it is within the self that spirituality is expressed and experienced. The self encompasses one's being (the essence of who one is), one's knowing (what one knows and how one knows), one's doing (the actions of living), and one's inner strength. However, it is not the self in isolation. Rather, the self-in-relationship or the self-connecting enfleshes spirituality. Caring connections with self, others, nature, and God or Universal Force shape the context within which, and through which, one's spirituality is experienced. I will illustrate my discussion primarily with references to the connectedness with nature. However, because of the unity of the experience, the other connections will become evident. Let me start by illustrating connection with Universal Force through others and nature.

CONNECTING WITH UNIVERSAL FORCE THROUGH OTHERS AND NATURE

Stories of various life experiences were used by participants as ways of illustrating their understandings of spirituality. The events recounted included times alone and times with others. Some stories made reference to God or Higher Power, and to religious practices. However, a distinction was made between religion and spirituality. When rituals or rules were important, they were viewed in relation to "something bigger than oneself," and in relation to how they helped one to live a better life. The women spoke of personal beliefs, not dogma, and included as general rules things such as loving, caring about others and the earth, doing for others, and ethical approaches to life.

God was mentioned in the context of church or religion, but was not limited to this context. Church, ministers, and ritual were addressed in terms of community and quality of relationship. Going to church was described in terms of connecting with communities in which one felt safe and experienced caring relationships more than in terms of beliefs and expectations in relationship to God. IH illustrated this when she described her experience of leaving her hometown and church to go to college:

I discovered that what was really most important is that community of people that I'd been a part of . . . more than what was the material, was the community itself, and that was what gave me the pleasure I got from going to church.

Some described a sense of connectedness with a Higher Power which was not necessarily named God. BB stated it this way:

Well, to me spirituality is being connected to everything and knowing that it goes beyond every person to something much bigger than all of us together, includes all of us. Growing up it was God, this entity out there. I don't believe that any more, but I do believe there is definitely a higher power of some sort.... We're all connected to this higher power ... we can call on it for a lot of healing and giving of healing and that kind of thing ... it's the one connector of everybody.

For DP, spirituality "means a connectedness to the universe and a sense that you have purpose here . . . a feeling that all of it is one substance." She reflected on the meaning of this connectedness, saying that "as I get to know those parts, those beings, creatures, whatever, then I will realize that I am much more like them than I am different from them." HC talked about what a "connection between God or a Higher Power" meant: "When I get up in the morning I'm thankful because I realize there is something that's making this world go around. . . . I think it's God. . . . I think it relates to the universe, the stars. . . . I just think that we're all connected." EG described deciding "probably this minute about whether there's God or not, cause I think there might be . . . it may be more of just a force that . . . looks over the whole universe, sort of oversees what's happening."

Participants described things like meditation, prayer, visualization, being in nature, ritual, reading the Bible and other books, and connecting with other people "in a higher way" as ways of connecting with the Higher Power. These might be done alone or with a group. In talking about her experiences of meditation and visualization, one participant stated, "When I visualize or when I meditate, all imaged energy is universal energy coming from above and below, and then I also believe I can send it out." Another participant talked about her daily walks as quiet times in which she reflects on passages from a book of daily meditations for women. Several participants talked about being more aware of their spirituality "outside, usually in connection with the earth."

FEEDING THE SPIRIT—CONNECTING WITH NATURE

Connecting with nature was a way in which participants fed or nurtured their spirits. When participants talked about their understandings of spirituality, they spoke of things like being outside, connecting with the earth, and deriving strength from nature. For some, there was something special about being in the mountains; others described experiences of the ocean, or spoke of activities and awarenesses related to things in nature such as gardening and appreciation of flowers. Connecting with the goddess was described by one participant as part of her spirituality, which helped her to appreciate the earth energy and become grounded.

EG discussed a time in her life when she was discovering more about what she valued. She talked about "finding how much it meant to me . . . just being surrounded by the mountains . . . the way it feels to be part of the earth here was what was making me think more about . . . a global picture of spirituality." She described finding "strength from either looking outside or being there and going places outside and being on the earth." She mentioned talking to the birds and thanking them for their singing, as a way of praying. For BB, doing ritual with a group is "essential in some way to spirituality" and acknowledges both each other and the earth changes. She noted that "the earth has really helped me appreciate that energy and get grounded . . . to be more congruent in my life." CV, BB, and DP all spoke of spending time in their gardens and close to the earth.

Being "outside," "in nature," "close to the earth" brought some of the participants more in touch with their spirituality. DP noted that "the times that I feel most spiritual are when I am alone and when I'm outside and walking or sitting . . . it happens outside usually in connection to the earth or the sun." GK talked about her awareness of the earth as "the big base," noting that it affected her, and stating that "being outside, being in touch with the earth . . . really is critical." When IH was speaking about situations in which she felt able to be free of some of the pulls and distractions in life, she said that "usually for me it's nature; I'm much more at home in the country and outside as opposed to inside. So then you get a sense of elevation from all those things that hold you down, and you get a sense of rising and being bigger."

Some of the participants mentioned that being near water, particularly the ocean, helped them to become more aware of their spirituality. IH stated that, for years, "going to the ocean was the biggest pleasure, physically, for me. It really gave me a sense of freedom and a sense of elation . . . anytime I'm around a body of water . . . it's that sense of peace and elation together." HC described experiences at the ocean and at a river in the following way:

> *When I'm at the ocean . . . I could sit there all day long . . . .*
> *I guess the water just does something to me. It just like*
> *calms me . . . you just feel freer . . . . I guess maybe when*
> *we were small my mother used to take us down to the river*
> *. . . and we'd be playing and it just seemed like it's so calm-*
> *ing. Whenever something bad happened, you go down*
> *there and everything was okay for the moment . . . and the*
> *ocean, it's so big, and just the sound, just walking on the*
> *sand or sitting there at the sunset is just beautiful . . . be-*
> *cause after I come back it's like I'm a new person . . . I feel*
> *alive again.*

APPRECIATE, RESPECT, CARE FOR NATURE

Appreciating, respecting, and caring for nature and the earth were described by participants as ways of expressing their spirituality. EG stated that "trying to respect the earth, since it's so important to me, may be a way that I express spirituality." IH told of devoting a lot of time to flowers: "I'll go around the country picking wild flowers and I decorate with them a lot; that's the main thing I do to decorate—to bring in flowers, even in the winter." BB and FE both talked about composting and recycling. FE also spoke of "a certain respect for the plants and for the wildlife" which she had learned from her father, and which she saw evident in her daughter's excitement over the blooming of a white violet that she had planted.

RELATIONSHIP WITH SELF IN CONNECTION WITH OTHERS AND NATURE

As noted previously, connectedness with self included one's being, one's knowing, one's doing, and one's inner strength. The sense of strength from nature was illustrated above. At the risk of being repetitious, I will give brief examples here of being, knowing, and doing in relationship to others and nature.

Being.   One participant described being when she said, "Spirituality is what is inside me, the way I express myself. It's just who I am." Another illustrated experiencing being in a "poignant moment that I have in my memory of having just run and come home, being in the bathtub with sunlight coming in and just being so totally in that moment, being relaxed and at peace and feeling the sun." Another described an experience during a process of esoteric healing in which "for that moment in time I was right in that place of just allowing and being, and it's hard to just be." EG talked about her need for "being outside . . . in nature and appreciating it." Others spoke of appreciating flowers, being in touch with the earth, and the need for being outside. In describing her experiences of the ocean HC stated, "I could sit there all day," just being there was soothing for her.

Knowing.   Knowing was reflected in an active seeking to learn about self and other things, as well as through intuitive awarenesses. Participants expressed an awareness of being connected to others, to a Universal Force, and to nature. A sense of inner knowing or trust in God was described by several of the women: "Just a strong belief in God . . . has helped me through it." "Just knowing I put all my faith and trust in Him . . . , He's always there." Another participant expressed the sense that there is "a force that looks over the whole universe, sort of oversees what's happening."

BB voiced an "understanding that we're all connected because we all have souls or higher selves." For DP, learning about different animals and other cultures brought the realization "that I am much more like them than I am different . . . people are pretty much the same." GK recognized that "in loving my children in that naked, raw, early mother-love . . . I saw . . . a piece of me that I wanted to grow." For EG, "just being surrounded by the mountains . . . was making me think more about the global picture."

Doing.   The women spoke of learning more about their connectedness with the earth and things of nature. This led them to take the time to be outside, to appreciate flowers and wildlife, to cultivate and care for gardens. It led to activities such as recycling and composting. DP illustrated this when she said, "because of that realization that you are connected and like other things, you tend to want to preserve those things and not bring any harm to them, to protect them."

SPIRITUALITY—LIVING OUR INTERCONNECTEDNESS

This section addresses spirituality in terms of living our interconnectedness. The awareness that spirituality incorporates interconnectedness, which was expressed by the women in this study, is similar to teachings of various ages and traditions. Their appreciation of a sense of connectedness was congruent with thoughts expressed by Hildegard of Bingen—everything in the world has been arranged by God in consideration of everything else and everything "in the heavens, on the earth, and under the earth, is penetrated with connectedness, is penetrated with relatedness" (quoted by Fox, 1985, p. 76). Their stories reflected what Carol Ochs (1983) noted, in her book *Women and Spirituality:* as "we come to identify with more and more of our world by knowing through being, we become more and more related to all of reality" (p. 141), and "through our relationship to people we can find the most ready access to a spiritual life" (p. 15).

The experiences of spirituality described here are echoed by Anderson and Hopkins (1991) in *The Feminine Face of God.* Their interviews with over 100 women indicated that, for women, spirituality implies relationship that connects. This relationship includes an opening to the sacred space within, making community, and connection to the earth. It is recognized that interconnected-ness is bittersweet, and includes both joy and pain, fullness and emptiness.

NURTURING SPIRIT

What can we learn from all of this about how to nurture spirit with ourselves and others? Let me preface these suggestions by saying again that a qualitative study with 12 women is not, in and of itself, a solid enough basis from which to make the leap to changes in nursing practice. The basis from which I make these suggestions is this study coupled with findings of other studies that described spirituality in similar ways (Anderson & Hopkins, 1991; Barker, 1989; Burkhardt, 1993; Hungelmann, Kenkel-Rossi, Klassen, & Stollenwerk, 1985). One other disclaimer is that this model is derived from women's understandings of spirituality, and still needs to be tested with men.

Spirit is the source of spirituality. Spirituality incorporates and is affected by one's experiences of living and by one's cosmology or worldview. A cosmology that adheres to directives such as having dominion over and subduing the earth suggests the possibility that earth is an object that can be exploited for one's own gains. When dominion is understood in terms of stewardship, the relationship changes to one of care. And a cosmology that views the earth as a living organism in which spirit lives in all beings provides a basis for knowing our interconnectedness with all of life. A reawakening to this latter worldview, I believe, is essential to the healing of ourselves and our world. This cosmology is reflected in Alice Walker's book, *The Color Purple* (1982). When the main characters, Celie and Shug, are talking about not being able to relate to the image of God presented to them in church, Shug says:

My first step from the old white man was trees. Then air. Then birds. Then other people. But one day when I was sitting quiet and feeling like a motherless child, which I was, it come to me: that feeling of being a part of everything, not separate at all. I knew that if I cut a tree, my arm would bleed. And I laughed and I cried and I run all around the house I knew just what it was. In fact, when it happen, you can't miss it. (p. 203)

Once we become aware of the elements of spirituality and the ways it is expressed and experienced, we can begin to recognize that, at some level, we have all been dealing with spirit in our nursing practice, but may not have been calling it by name. Part of our reawakening is naming the experience. It is important to develop ways of nurturing spirit within ourselves and others in order to expand our ability to recognize and incorporate spirituality in our care with others.

The women in this study are our teachers regarding ways of nurturing spirit. The first lesson is that we must *listen.* This may mean reawakening, with awareness of spirit, that part of our own spirit that hears. We must listen first within ourselves, and pay attention to the spirit or sacred space within. From this place, we can listen more attentively to others, hearing their spirits and learning about their spiritualities. In this process, it is good to be reminded of the secret the fox shared with the Little Prince: "It is only with the heart that one can see rightly; what is essential is invisible to the eye" (Saint-Exupéry, 1971, p. 87).

Listening is something that may come more easily for some than for others; in either case, it takes practice. Making time and space to "be" with oneself is a good beginning. In this process, we can pay attention to where one's being is drawn and nurtured. This might be done through prayer, meditation, visualization, a warm bath, walking outside, sitting at the ocean, listening to music, or meaningful reading. Appreciating and valuing oneself, feeling love and unity with friends and family, and experiencing connection with nature are ways of being.

Spirit is nurtured through processes of learning about who one is, one's mission, what matters in life, and one's connections with God/others/nature. At times, this is done by looking at one's life in retrospect to see the patterns that have been unfolding; recognizing times of adversity as opportunities for growth and spiritual awakening; paying attention to one's inner senses and learning to trust one's own experiences. This can be done through such things as reading about gardening, talking to a friend about how to grow certain plants, or planting and letting the plant be the teacher. Reminiscing is one way to review one's life and discover patterns; counseling is another. Journaling may be useful when one is seeking to know the self better. Paying attention to physical symptoms and reactions can be another source of insight.

Nurturing spirit requires doing those things that nurture one's connectedness. Connecting with God or Universal Force might mean participation in religious activities, Bible study, learning about one's traditions, walking outside, or quietly observing a sunset. Cultivating, preserving, and caring for the earth through composting, gardening, or recycling; choosing to live more simply; working for clean rivers and air; or just spending time outdoors are ways of connecting with nature. Relationships with family and others include activities such as extending love and care, spending time together, sharing joys and pains, passing on heritage and traditions, connecting with ancestors, and providing for needs. Connection with self includes acknowledging one's worth, taking care of physical needs through exercise and healthful diet, allowing quiet time for self-renewal, writing poetry, walking, and engaging in personal growth work.

Facilitating nurture of spirit with others requires knowing the important connections and what is meaningful in those persons' lives. Listening for cues and aiding someone in naming the connections may be helpful. Frequently, this can be done by just giving the person an opportunity to talk about what is important. (Several women in my study commented that they were so glad to have been asked about spirituality; no one had ever asked them about this before!)

An interview itself becomes an intervention. If a person is hospitalized, or homebound, and unable to be outside, connecting with nature may be done through visualization, bringing pictures of a garden, listening to nature-sounds tapes, reminiscing about working in a garden in the past, and having plants around. Perhaps the custom of sending flowers to those who are hospitalized or homebound reflects the need for staying connected. Rituals such as daily prayer, meditation, walking, or listening to relaxation tapes can be very useful for people dealing with stress and situational anxiety.

This list can go on and on, but space is limited. Anderson and Hopkins (1991) suggested that spiritual unfolding may be likened to a sacred garden that can be entered through many gates. Persons may go through these entry points in a variety of ways at different times in their lives. The key for nursing is to recognize that all persons we encounter manifest spirituality in their own unique ways. With each process of spiritual unfolding, our role is to identify, with the person, the gate or gates that are being utilized at that time. More concretely, let me suggest some questions that may facilitate the process of discovering the gates for yourselves and with others:

What are the important connections and things that bring meaning within your own life?

If connecting with a Universal Force or God is important, how do you do this? Where and when have you felt this connection most clearly? Is prayer a part of this connection?

What is prayer to you? If you pray or meditate, where do you do this? with whom? Do you need to speak words, or is being still enough?

Where do you find that you connect better—in a church or temple? In the sacred space of nature? Walking? Sitting? In your home?

How do you express prayer—through words? silence? or in an active way such as dancing, playing music, tending a garden, caring for family, cooking, reading? Is ritual involved, with others or alone, such as religious services, chanting, drumming, lighting candles, preparing the soil to plant, preparing a special meal?

What helps you when you are frightened? worried? hurting? lonely? sad? Do you feel a need for being by yourself to sort things out, or do you seek the presence of others?

How do you discover your own inner wisdom and inner strength? With whom would you want to connect during these times? Where do you find comfort? What activities are helpful?

What activities, things, and places bring you pleasure and joy? (It has been said that a happy heart is God's greatest gift.)

What excites you? When do you feel your spirit lifted? Where do you feel most alive—at the ocean? in the desert? in the mountains? listening to music? dancing? at the birth of a child? with certain persons? during prayer or meditation?

Who are the important persons in your life? What are your special memories with these persons? When you are together, where do you like to be? What do you like to do?

How have your relationships developed through pleasant and unpleasant times? How have you cultivated these relationships? What nurtures the relationships when distance is between you? How do you express care for the persons in these relationships?

What relationships have been difficult, and how have you grown through these experiences?

What have you learned from your elders/ancestor, and what do you want to pass on to the children you know? How do you pass on what is important to you?

What do you do to take care of yourself? What is life-giving and inspiriting for you?

What is your story? What would be the titles of the chapters in the book of your life? What chapter are you in now?

What do you do to care for the earth? How do you appreciate and understand your connection with the earth and nature?

Living our connectedness is crucial to helping others in living theirs. In a speech attributed to Chief Seattle, we can find some insights into the process of living our interconnectedness with all of life. I close with parts of this speech, adapted from the renditions found in *Brother Eagle, Sister Sky* (Jeffers, 1991) and *The Power of Myth* (Campbell, 1988).

Every part of this earth is sacred to my people. If we sell you our land you must remember that it is sacred. The perfumed flowers are our sisters. The bear, deer, great eagle are our brothers. We all belong to the same family. All things are connected. What are we without the beasts? If the beasts were gone, we would die from a great loneliness of spirit. We are part of the earth and the earth is part of us. The earth is precious to God. To harm the earth is to heap contempt on its

*Creator. The earth does not belong to us, we belong to the
earth. All things are connected like the blood that unites one
family. We do not weave the web of life, we are but a strand
in the web. What we do to the web we do to ourselves. The
earth is our mother. What befalls the earth befalls the sons
and daughters of the earth. Preserve the land for all children, loving it as God loves us all.*

PERSONAL STATEMENT

It is hard to say when my interest in the environment began. My
early experiences in Girl Scouting and camping gave me an appreciation for being in nature. More conscious awareness of my
connectedness with all of life emerged through my experiences in
and after college. Understanding health as being in harmony with
nature was a lesson that I learned through my work as a public
health nurse with the Navajo people. Native American teachings
continue to help me to recognize that I am part of the interdependent web of life. This leads me to realize that what I do and
how I act affects not only my immediate environment, but the
earth as a whole. A friend recently wrote: "As I believe, so I behave. As I behave, so I become. As I become, so becomes my
world." Because of this knowledge, I choose to do things such as
garden, be outside frequently, recycle, compost, buy in bulk when
possible so as to decrease trash in our landfills. I choose to avoid
red meat and to eat primarily vegetarian fare, not only because it
feels healthier, but because it is one response to world hunger. (It
takes a good deal more grain to feed cattle than to feed poultry,
and the rain forest might be less likely to be destroyed if the demand for beef were diminished.) Living in awareness is what I find
to be most important and difficult at the same time. This means appreciating that the air I breathe is touched by the breath of people
thousands of miles away, as well as by the trees, plants, birds, animals, and so on. It means recognizing that my thoughts and feelings send out energy that affects all in my environment, and that
attending to my own growth, well-being, transformation, and healing contributes to the healing of our world. Attentiveness to my

spiritual being is essential for me in this process. My interest in environmental concerns is sustained by the awareness that I am part of a living organism that we call Mother Earth, and I can no more ignore what is happening to the environment than I could an imbalance in my own body.

REFERENCES

Anderson, S. R., & Hopkins, P. (1991). *The feminine face of God.* New York: Bantam Books.

Barker, E. R. (1989). *Spiritual well-being in Appalachian women.* Unpublished doctoral dissertation, University of Texas, Austin.

Burkhardt, M. A. (1989). Spirituality: An analysis of the concept. *Holistic Nursing Practice, 3*(3), 69–77.

Burkhardt, M. A. (1993). Characteristics of spirituality in the lives of women in a rural Appalachian community. *Journal of Transcultural Nursing, 4*(2), 19–23.

Burkhardt, M. A., & Nagai-Jacobson, M. G. (1994). Reawakening spirit in clinical practice. *Journal of Holistic Nursing, 12*(1), 9–21.

Campbell, J. (1988). *The power of myth.* New York: Doubleday.

Carson, V. B. (1989). *Spiritual dimensions of nursing practice.* Philadelphia: Saunders.

Clifford, M., & Gruca, A. (1987). Facilitating spiritual care in the rehabilitation setting. *Rehabilitation Nursing, 12*(6), 131–159.

Fox, M. (1985). *Illuminations of Hildegard of Bingen.* Santa Fe, NM: Bear & Company.

Glaser, B. G., & Strauss, A. L. (1967). *Discovery of grounded theory: Strategies for qualitative research.* New York: Aldine.

Green, R. (1986). Healing and spirituality. *The Practitioner, 1422*(230), 1087–1093.

Hungelmann, J., Kenkel-Rossi, E., Klassen, L., & Stollenwerk, R. M. (1985). Spiritual well-being in older adults: Harmonious interconnectedness. *Journal of Religion and Health, 24*(2), 147–153.

Jeffers, S. (1991). *Brother eagle, sister sky.* New York: Dial Books.

Lincoln, Y. S., & Guba, E. G. (1985). *Naturalistic inquiry.* Beverly Hills, CA: Sage.

Mickley, J. R., Soeken, K., & Belcher, A. (1992). Spiritual well-being, religiousness and hope among women with breast cancer. *Image: The Journal of Nursing Scholarship, 24*(4), 267–272.

Nagai-Jacobson, M. G., & Burkhardt, M. A. (1989). Spirituality: Cornerstone of holistic nursing practice. *Holistic Nursing Practice, 3*(3), 18–26.

Ochs, C. (1983). *Women and spirituality.* Totowa, NJ: Rowman & Allenheld.

Saint-Exupéry, A. (1971). *The little prince.* New York: Harcourt Brace Jovanovich.

Siegel, B. (1986). *Love, medicine, and miracles.* New York: Harper & Row.

Stiles, M. K. (1990). The shining stranger: Nurse–family spiritual relationship. *Cancer Nursing, 13*(4), 235–245.

Stuart, E. M., Deckro, J. P., & Mandle, C. L. (1989). Spirituality in health and healing: A clinical program. *Holistic Nursing Practice, 3*(3), 35–46.

Walker, A. (1982). *The color purple.* New York: Pocket Books.

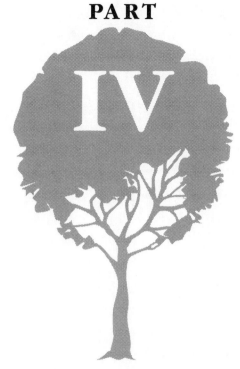

Nursing's Accountability to the Future

This concluding part presents a composite view of ways nurses and organizations enact environmental accountability. We present these perspectives as a way of stimulating your thoughts and creativity about how you might live your own commitment to environmental accountability.

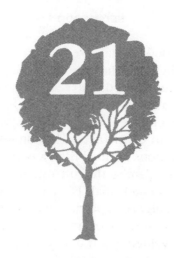

An Ecofeminist Look at
Animal Research

Betsy Todd

*Look into the eyes of an animal. As you look into those eyes,
reflect that this being is a never-to-be-duplicated expression
of the universe. Pay attention to what you see: the years of
living present within those eyes, and the vitality that shines
through their color and transparency. Pay attention also to
what you cannot see, the inwardness, the selfhood, the "I"
that is as singular as its outward expression. What you look
upon is a living spirit. Greet and respect it. Appreciate it for
what it is.*

—Kowalski (1991, pp. 91–92)

very *hour,* 20,000 animals are killed in the world's research labs. Before they die, they are irradiated, shocked, burned, drowned, dismembered, starved, blinded, paralyzed, and shot. They are separated from their mothers at birth; ripped from their families in the wild; kept in isolation for years; battered with pistons and whirled in centrifuges. How should people who understand our connections with all life view these facts?

Some readers may dismiss this introduction to the subject as "unprofessional" and emotional. For many, the influence of the Western science paradigm and patriarchal "rationality" is so strong that these are seen as soft, "womanish" concerns. What is called science is so highly valued that it overshadows thoughtful consideration of multidimensional scientific issues. Not surprisingly, then, as nurses (striving for acceptance as scientific professionals) and as individuals, our relationship to animal research goes largely unexamined.

Since the 17th century, animal experimentation has been promoted as central to medical research efforts. The idea of using other animals as surrogates for people is intuitively appealing, and the experiments themselves are dramatic manipulations of other living creatures. Yet once we circumvent the elaborate, man[sic]made system of assumptions, and the "proofs" that claim to support its value and necessity, the scientific and ethical limitations of animal research become clear.

HISTORICAL PERSPECTIVES

The Baconian/Cartesian school of scientific thought has shaped the traditions of Western medical research. Bacon (1561–1626) asserted that true knowledge is attained only when the object of study can be isolated and manipulated in a controlled laboratory setting. To Bacon, the scientist is one who must "torture Nature's secrets from her." According to Descartes (1596–1650), animals are machines that can be broken apart and studied, piece by piece, to learn about whole organisms.

These perspectives are the foundation of modern scientific thought. They "stand in stark contrast to that aspect of traditional,

Aristotelian science that calls for observation immersed in natural context as the way to comprehend, in its totality, the essential nature of that which is observed" (Freeman & Mensch, 1989, p. 36).

This unholistic worldview is the basis for a medical research paradigm characterized by reductionism, dominance/control, and measurability. These constitute what Phillips (1993) called "the process by which scientific 'facts' are socially created." In other words, Baconian/Cartesian thought about what constitutes the "valid" path to knowledge is a societal construct, not a universal truth. Unfortunately, this legacy has made it difficult to explore illness, medicine, and animal experimentation from an integrated and holistic perspective.

The influence of these ideas—never without opposition from scientists with different worldviews—has led to more than 300 years of animal experiments. Sir George Pickering, of Oxford, England, has commented on the scientific fashion that continues to this day:

> *The idea, as I understand it, is that fundamental truths are revealed in laboratory experiments on lower [sic] animals and are then applied to the problems of the sick patient. Having been myself trained as a physiologist [and physician], I feel in a way competent to assess such a claim. It is plain nonsense. (1964, p. 1616)*

As animal experimentation became firmly entrenched in scientific circles, major advances in public health were also taking place. Improved sanitation and nutrition, literacy campaigns, and higher standards of living resulted in a healthier populace. Remarkably, the animal experimenters took credit for these changes, claiming that the value of their "modern laboratory science" was confirmed by the public's better health. Medical historians have disagreed, and have exposed the experimenters' claims as blatantly false revisionist history.

McKeown wrote:

> *Those who look mainly to laboratory research for the solution of current health problems do so under some mis-*

*apprehensions about its achievements in the past. They un-
derestimate the part that has been played by a rising standard of living and the accompanying advances in literacy,
and they overestimate the contribution of laboratory medicine. (1976, p. 145)*

The events of recent decades provide continuing evidence of
the failure of animal experiments to contribute to medical
progress. Since President Nixon declared the War on Cancer in
1970, billions of dollars and millions of animal lives have been "invested" in the effort. The result: the age-adjusted incidence and
mortality rates for cancer have *increased* by 8.5% and 8.7%, respectively (Bailar & Smith, 1986). Animal "models" have been a
central focus of AIDS research as well; yet, virtually all of our
knowledge of HIV and AIDS has come from clinical and epidemiological work, autopsies, and *in vitro* studies (Todd, 1991). Clinical and epidemiological studies, not animal experiments, have
formed the basis for current recommendations about diet, exercise, and life-style changes in the prevention of heart disease.

ANIMAL RESEARCH:
SCIENCE VERSUS BELIEF SYSTEM

Whether the subjects of a study are mice, rats, dogs, cats, horses,
chimpanzees, or any other nonhuman animal, they will differ from
humans anatomically and physiologically. This makes the extrapolation of data from one species to another extremely unreliable.
Knowing what we do about the great variability in, for example,
drug effects among people of different ages, genders, genetic back-
grounds, and states of health, it should come as no surprise that *interspecies* variations are at least as significant. (Interestingly,
women have pointed out for years that research on men is irrele-
vant to women's health; yet the power of the Western science paradigm is such that inter*species* variability is rarely discussed.)

There are certainly biological similarities between humans and
other animals, but the parallels are too superficial to allow detailed analogies to be drawn between species. Sameness that

seemed significant three centuries ago—four limbs, skeletal similarities, a beating heart, a brain with two hemispheres—are seen today as woefully inadequate bases on which to draw conclusions about complex living organisms.

Data from other animals are difficult to assess not only because of these basic interspecies differences in immunity, metabolism, biochemistry, and so on, but also because experimental variables are routinely uncontrolled (Barnard & Hou, 1988); numbers are often statistically insignificant (especially in primate studies); and the role of cofactors—such as diet, exercise, drug use, environmental pollution, and stress—in the development of disease is entirely ignored.

In discussing the science of animal research with high school students, I often present them with the following scenarios:

1. You are a scientist who wants to learn about heartworm, a dangerous and often fatal infection in dogs. Your lab works primarily with cats, however, so you design a feline heartworm study. This involves injecting cats with heartworm and collecting data on their response to experimental drugs.

2. You want to learn about beards—what determines the onset of facial hair growth, and why some men have thicker beards than others. But because your university is a women's institution, your only potential research subjects are women. Your study design, approved by the university's human subjects review committee, involves injecting female volunteers with "male" hormones that will induce facial hair growth.

These manipulations are precisely the kinds of "scientific" interventions that are the basis of animal experiments. High school students have not yet internalized mainstream science assumptions about the accuracy of experimentally induced diseases or interspecies extrapolation, yet these teenagers readily point out the scientific limitations of these proposals. "Cats don't naturally acquire heartworm, so it can't be exactly the same disease. . . . A cat won't metabolize drugs in the same way a dog will. . . . A woman's beard will not be the same as a man's. . . . Hormones will cause other changes that may affect the study results." And so on.

If animal "models" of disease and injury were designed today, they would never be taken seriously by the scientific community. An elaborate belief system, promoted by those with a vested interest in the dominance/control paradigm and reinforced by the public's fear of disease and death, supports the scientifically flawed idea that experiments on nonhuman animals are the key to medical progress.

EMOTIONS, ETHICS, AND ANIMAL EXPERIMENTS

Although the scientific illogic of animal experimentation is enough to compel many of us to reject this methodology, there are other ways of knowing that can deepen our understanding of this issue. Theologian Andrew Linzey has spoken of "a knowing that comes through empathy and communion" (Arbogast, 1993, p. 15). A "felt experience" is a particularly significant way of knowing for women (see Bateson, 1990; Gilligan, 1982), but it is repeatedly de-legitimatized by dominant norms of "rational" (male) thought.

Animals who end their lives in a research lab are no different from other nonhuman animals we know. In the meditation at the beginning of this chapter, Kowalski makes the point with great reverence: each animal is an individual whose life is important to him or her. Yet these fellow beings are regarded by many as "tools" of research. They are "highly specialized scientific instruments" (Phillips, 1993) or "part instrument, part reagent, a complicated and incidentally sentient system" (Lane-Petter, 1963, pp. vii–viii).

Collard (1988) wrote:

> *The researcher strips the animal of its natural attributes and manipulates it to suit his design. The animal no longer exudes grace, strength, and health. Restricted in body and mind, and drastically altered, it [sic] is afflicted with physical and mental diseases. . . . As the animal is forcibly alienated from [her] essence and isolated from [her] kin, so [she] is separated from the researcher. (p. 58)*

According to patriarchal science, we are not supposed to feel connected to these animals. In a society grounded in hierarchical differences, we must regard these creatures as separate from us, rather than as varying and joyous expressions of a larger whole. Seeing them as "other" makes it easier to deny the animals' experiences. Then, *against our intuitive judgment,* we accept the researchers' claims that torturing animals is a scientific necessity rather than a terrible act of violence.

Most of us can empathize with the sufferings of one animal, but the knowledge that millions are suffering leaves us numb. Heyward (1993) wondered whether "we trivialize the fate of nonhuman animals *not* because we don't think their lives are important but because we *know* it's all connected, and we are simply overwhelmed" (p. 8).

It is, of course, scientific blasphemy to bring up the animals' experience. This is "subjective" (as though such a thing as scientific objectivity exists), "unprofessional," unscientific. Such attempts to label (and thereby marginalize) a decidedly "womanish" viewpoint is only one of the strategies employed by science to deflect thoughtful discussion of the realities of animal experimentation. Five other techniques are used regularly to manipulate public perceptions of medical research: (1) locating reality, (2) framing the issue, (3) naming, (4) institutionalizing technology, and (5) setting social priorities. Each is discussed here in turn.

Locating Reality

Like the Church hierarchy before them, scientists consider themselves arbiters of reality for the masses. The Baconian idea that something is true only if it can be proven in a laboratory makes the laboratory, not life, the center of knowledge and the focus of attention. Griffin (1989) described this perspective as one in which "ideas, words, numbers, concepts have become more real to this mind than material reality" (p. 13). As noted above, this is an artificial construct that serves particular societal ends.

The idea of animal laboratory work as some kind of gold standard in medical research promotes disinformation about more useful and practical work such as epidemiology and human clinical studies. Animal researchers would have us believe that these real-world methods are somehow speculative or subjective.

Framing the Issue

The public is led to believe that the only questions to be asked about animal research involve animal welfare. The underlying faulty premise on which this work is based—the idea that animal experiments can somehow reveal truths about human health and illness—is thus not exposed to public scrutiny.

In addition, the choice to do animal research is framed as being between saving human lives or saving animal lives. The implication is that either animals must be harmed or the quality of medical care will plummet. Bill Moyer of the Social Movement Empowerment Project calls this kind of strategy the creation of a societal myth. In reality, animal experiments harm both animals and people—animals very directly and acutely, and humans because this nonscientific methodology squanders resources that could be better spent on more productive research, prevention, and treatment. The actual dichotomy here is between the public's health and the vested interests of a powerful biomedical elite.

Naming

Any powerful group uses language to reinforce the status quo from which it profits. Vivisection becomes known as "biomedical research"; pain is "reaction to aversive stimuli"; animals are "sacrificed," not killed; the Cruelty to Animals Act governing animal experiments in Britain is replaced by the Animals (Scientific Procedures) Act.

Institutionalizing Technology

Some animal "models" of disease are technologically quite amazing. The manipulations involved in producing SCID-hu mice that harbor human immune cells, or transgenic animals with "cystic fibrosis," are remarkable and costly, and these models are seen to have such value that their inapplicability to human disease is obscured.

Setting Social Priorities

A disproportionate emphasis on medical "cures" ensures steady research funding at the expense of treatment and prevention programs. Relevant medical research *is* important, but even research without animals should not take precedence over treating the sick or preventing illness and injury. Yet, the glories of research endeavors consistently outdraw mundane (and less expensive) prevention and education activities—a fact painfully obvious during the current AIDS pandemic.

In addition, the emphasis on animal experimentation as "hard" science (an interesting patriarchal adjective, with its connotations of superior, more effectual, more potent) guarantees that epidemiology, clinical studies, and extraordinary new *in vitro* technologies (three-dimensional cell cultures, for example) will be underfunded and underused.

On the subject of animal experimentation, mainstream science has managed to control public perceptions of ongoing work just as it has controlled the animals in their labs. We must break out of the confines of what we are told about medical research, and begin to see the realities of patriarchal science. Only then can we work for change.

No animal, large or small, has evolved biologically and psychically to be used as a living tool; to fulfill its destiny in tanks and cages, strapped to experimental chairs and tables; to further man's causes and help him devise ways to cure his mental and physical disorders. Disease and neuroses are human problems. Progress is a human obsession. No animal has played a role in these disorders. No animal is responsible for them. And no amount of animal research will correct them. (Collard, 1988, p. 66)

PERSONAL STATEMENT

I was "always" an environmentalist, but it wasn't until I listened more closely to other-than-human animals that certain facts began to resonate with me. A flyer announcing an animal rights demonstration got me started. I read its description of a research project that seemed cruel, useless, and frankly unbelievable to a person like me, schooled in mainstream science. My nursing background pushed me to investigate (what are we nurses, if not seekers of justice, and committed to lifelong learning??), and I soon found myself allied with other health workers in the Medical Research Modernization Committee (New York) and the Physicians Committee for Responsible Medicine (Washington, DC). Both groups oppose animal experiments, and they guided my exploration of the medical literature on the subject.

It was the Feminists for Animal Rights (FAR), however, that put it all together for me. FAR (Chapel Hill, NC) works to raise consciousness about the connections between sexism and speciesism in a patriarchal society. FAR members are ecofeminists, concerned about the devaluation and destruction of nature and the earth.

I'm sustained in my daily commitment to animals and the earth by a vegetarian diet, which respects all animal life (including my own) and helps me tread more lightly on the planet.

REFERENCES

Arbogast, M. (1993). Reclaiming a positive tradition: Interview with Andrew Linzey. *The Witness, 76*(10), 15–18.

Bailar, J. C., & Smith, E. M. (1986). Progress against cancer. *New England Journal of Medicine, 314,* 1226–1232.

Barnard, N., & Hou, S. (1988, September). Inherent stress: The tough life in lab routine. *Lab Animal, 17*(6), 21–27.

Bateson, M. C. (1990). *Composing a life.* New York: Plume/Penguin Books.

Collard, A. (1988). *Rape of the wild.* Bloomington: Indiana University Press.

Freeman, A., & Mensch, B. (1989, September/October). Scratching the belly of the beast. *Tikkun, 4*(5), 34–38, 92–96.

Gilligan, C. (1982). *In a different voice.* Boston: Harvard University Press.

Griffin, S. (1989). Split culture. In J. Plant (Ed.), *Healing the wounds: The promise of ecofeminism.* Philadelphia: New Society Publishers.

Heyward, C. (1993). The bear and Bosnia. *The Witness, 76*(10), 15–18.

Kowalski, G. (1991). *The souls of animals* (pp. 91–92). New Hampshire: Stillpoint Publishing.

Lane-Petter, W. (Ed.). (1963). *Animals for research: Principles of breeding and management.* London: Academic Press.

McKeown, T. (1976). *The role of medicine: Dream, mirage, or nemesis?* London: Nuffield Provincial Hospitals Trust.

Phillips, M. T. (1994, Summer). Proper names and the social construction of biography: The negative case of laboratory animals. *Qualitative Sociology, 17*(2), 119–142.

Pickering, S. G. (1964). Physician and scientist. *British Medical Journal,* 1615–1618.

Todd, B. (1991). *Animal research and AIDS.* Unpublished Master's thesis. New York: Columbia University School of Public Health.

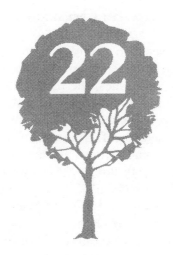

The Environment as a Curricular Concept in Professional Nursing Programs: A Case Study

Elisabeth A. Pennington

INTRODUCTION

Nursing has, for many years, acknowledged a metaparadigm that assists in the definition of professional nursing. The concepts of the metaparadigm are: man, health, environment, and nursing. These concepts help to define nursing, its role in society, and the scope of practice.

In the 1980s, prompted by accreditation criteria that required a conceptual framework, many schools of nursing engaged in major

*The author wishes to acknowledge the contributions of the Undergraduate Committee Task Force, University of Michigan, School of Nursing, who developed the revised curriculum of which this study is a part.

curricular revision based on a conceptual model. With many individuals attempting to come together with a variety of ideas, special interests, concerns, and issues, the responsibility of structuring knowledge for meaning is a daunting task. A conceptual base assists the process by providing both a focus and boundaries for the task. A conceptual base also facilitates internal consistency and logic in the design. Some schools attempted to utilize practice models (e.g., Orem, 1980; Roy, 1984); others used an "eclectic model," that is, their own definitions of these concepts.

The University of Michigan School of Nursing faculty, in 1987, determined that a curricular change was necessary. The conceptual base on which the curriculum would be built needed to focus on the client as the center of activity. The nurse's role would emphasize critical thinking, independent judgment, and clinical decision making. Many hours of discussion, reading, and serious thought were put into the conceptual design. Discussions regarding the faculty definitions and understanding of the metaparadigm concepts of man (humankind), health, and nursing were lively and creative, but the concept of environment proved to be the most challenging.

DEFINING THE ENVIRONMENT

A review of the concept of the environment in nursing was undertaken, using two approaches. The first was a review of how the concept was defined by the popular theorists of the day. The models of Erickson, Tomlin, and Swain (1983), Johnson (1980), King (1981), Neumann (1982), Orem (1980), Peplau (1952), Rogers (1970), and Roy (1984) were reviewed. Most of these theorists defined the environment broadly, indicating that the environment was "all of the forces external to the individual." A few also included the notion of "internal environments." Rogers (1970) presented a detailed and complex notion of the environment, but without the rest of her theoretical model it was not useful for this faculty. All theorists agreed that humans interact with the environment. The influence of the nurse on the environment was often inferred, but usually not explicitly addressed.

The second review was to sample how other professional schools of nursing dealt with this concept in their curricula design. A number of accreditation self-study reports were reviewed, as well as curricular documents obtained from a variety of programs. The majority of curricula indicated that the environment was "everything external to the individual." Some programs substituted "society" for environment. Many did not specifically define the environment but did include the notion that it affected client health.

The faculty of the University of Michigan felt strongly that the environment is a critical concept of the metaparadigm and is specifically connected to our professional history. The environment is part of the social mandate of nursing, as noted by the work, in the late 18th century and the 19th century, that focused on sanitation and hygiene (Novak, 1988). The growth of public health nursing was based on the need to address environmental factors and their negative impact on health. This historical link seemed more imperative than ever as the faculty considered the effects of air and water pollution, the destruction of the ozone layer, insecticides, poor education, inadequate housing, and crime.

The literature in nursing indicated that the environment raised practice issues. The impact of a particular environment on patient outcomes had been studied (e.g., Richardson, 1987), as had manipulation of the environment as a therapeutic technique (e.g., Whedon & Shedd, 1989). The faculty believed that the environment impacts the care of the chronically ill individual differently than the care of the acutely ill. The setting in which care takes place also impacts the care delivered and received.

Ultimately, the faculty agreed on the following definition of the environment:

The environment is comprised of all the external conditions, circumstances, and forces which influence, and are influenced by the client. The concept of the environment is broad and includes the following factors:

1. *The Physical Environment—physical properties, ecological concerns, population structures.*

2. *The Sociocultural Environment—legal, ethical, cultural, technological, political, economic and organizations.*

After this definition was determined, the faculty turned their attention to the role of nursing in relation to the environment. Additionally, there was concern that the definition was so broad that the student would need guidance in trying to focus and incorporate the concept into the role of the nurse. What would the faculty expect the student to learn and practice?

The following statement was added to the basic definition:

The nurse understands that the dynamic interaction between the client and the environment affects health and the achievement of health goals. The professional nurse considers the environment in relation to the client:

a. *The immediate and surrounding environment, both physical and psychosocial, which is critical in the immediate care of the client.*

b. *The contextual environment, which surround the immediate situation. Generally, this environment (both physical and psychosocial) is a contributor to the overall care of the client.*

c. *The potential environment, which influences the long-term health of the client and lays the foundation for health promotion activities.*

The professional nurse assesses the environment and is capable of modifying some aspects of the environment in order to enhance clients' wellness. Evaluation of nursing interventions also considers changes that may have occurred in the environment. (University of Michigan, 1989, p. 6)

Figure 22-1 presents a graphic representation of the curriculum concepts. The client is in the center, and has both wellness and illness needs in a number of identified dimensions. The "client" can be an individual, family, aggregate group, or community, and exists

Figure 22–1   Interaction of Curriculum Concepts

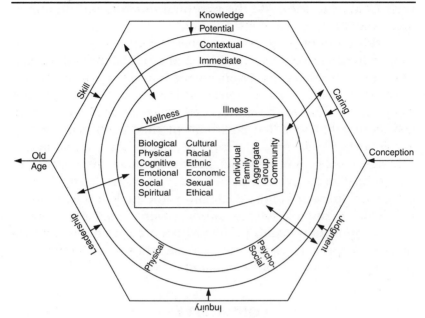

on an age continuum. Surrounding the client is the environment, which has both physical and psychosocial aspects. The outer frame illustrates the components of professional nursing. The arrows indicate nursing's influence on the environment, and, through the environment, on the client.

CONCEPT UTILIZATION

In this curriculum, environment is used both as a pervasive subconcept and as a progressive subconcept. As a pervasive subconcept, the physical and psychosocial environment is considered whenever a client's health status is being assessed. Modification of the environment is a factor in the planning of nursing care at every level of the curriculum.

As a progressive subconcept, attention is paid to the immediate, contextual, and potential environments. Assessment and interventions are focused, for the beginning student, on the client's immediate environment. As students progress through the curriculum, they consider the contextual environment. In their final year, they add the potential environment to assessment and intervention considerations.

As this concept progresses, so does the definition of client—from individual to family, and then to groups and the community. Thus, the student has experience with considering many aspects of the environment. For instance, in the fourth level of the curriculum, the focus is on wellness and the community as client. In considering the immediate environment, the student will conduct a community assessment, which includes data on population (physical), pollution (physical), health resources (psychosocial), educational levels (psychosocial), and so on. Considering the contextual environment of the community, the student might look at statewide or national policies and/or resources, and assess potential environmental health problems that are national or international in scope, such as the effects of migrant worker immigration patterns on the health of a community.

OBJECTIVES

Because the definition of the environment is broad and includes a number of content areas, it is referenced in many of the curriculum objectives. However, the faculty also believed that a specific curriculum objective was necessary to underscore the importance of this concept of the nursing metaparadigm. The curriculum objective is:

Identify, plan, and implement strategies to promote or modify environments which are sufficient to maintain and achieve desired outcomes.

This curriculum objective is further delineated into level objectives appropriate for the four levels of the curriculum. They are:

Level One   Understand the concept of the environment and its impact on health.

Level Two   Identify how an individual's environment can impact on his or her health status and on nursing outcomes.

Assess clients' immediate environment and identify specific variables that can be modified or altered to promote wellness.

Level Three   Plan and implement interventions that modify a client's immediate and contextual environment in order to promote wellness.

Level Four   Assess the environmental variables that affect a community's health.

Assess, plan, and implement interventions that modify a client's immediate, contextual, and potential environment in order to promote wellness.

OUTCOMES

The above objectives are clinical in nature. However, this concept is integrated in virtually every course, including nutrition, research, family concepts, nursing therapies, and especially in a fourth-level course, societal health issues. Here, students focus on issues such as poverty, violence, pollution, overpopulation, and life-styles. Thus, they have an opportunity to truly consider the potential environment and develop creative nursing strategies. Students take this course along with a professional development course that focuses on political action. The two make a great combination and foster activism in the students.

Students report that they feel well-equipped to consider a broad range of health issues and problems. Inclusion of both the physical and psychosocial environments forces students to focus beyond the medical model. Some state that they feel they have discovered nursing's "roots" because as they have searched the literature about a current problem, they have discovered the relevance of the work of such nursing luminaries as Florence Nightingale, Lillian Wald, and others.

The faculty feel that this curriculum prepares students to face the challenges of modern nursing. They have been exposed not only to environmental factors that affect health, but also to those factors that impinge on professional practice. Because of its uniqueness, inclusion of this concept has presented creative challenges to the faculty to provide learning experiences that are illustrative and helpful to the student. Further, as health care increasingly moves into community settings, this concept, perhaps more than the others, takes on particular importance. This faculty has built a sound base on which other experiences can be structured.

REFERENCES

Erickson, H. C., Tomlin, E. M., & Swain, M. A. (1983). *Modeling and role-modeling: A theory and paradigm for nursing.* Englewood Cliffs, NJ: Prentice-Hall.

Johnson, D. E. (1980). The behavioral system model for nursing. In J. P. Riehl & C. Roy (Eds.), *Conceptual models for nursing practice* (2nd ed.). New York: Appleton-Century-Crofts.

King, I. M. (1981). *A theory for nursing: Systems, concepts, process.* New York: Wiley.

Neumann, B. (1982). *The Neumann Systems Model: Application to nursing education and practice.* Norwalk, CT: Appleton-Century-Crofts.

Novak, J. C. (1988). The social mandate and historical basis for nursing's role in health promotion. *Journal of Professional Nursing, 4*(2), 80–87.

Orem, D. E. (1980). *Nursing: Concepts of practice.* New York: McGraw-Hill.

Peplau, H. E. (1952). *Interpersonal relations in nursing.* New York: Putnam.

Richardson, B. K. (1987). Psychiatric inpatients' perceptions of the seclusion-room experience. *Nursing Research, 36*(4), 234–238.

Rogers, M. E. (1970). *An introduction to the theoretical base of nursing.* Philadelphia: Davis.

Roy, C. (1984). *An introduction to nursing: An adaptation model* (2nd ed.). Englewood Cliffs, NJ: Prentice-Hall.

University of Michigan, School of Nursing Faculty. (1989). *Diversity in design: The undergraduate curriculum.* Ann Arbor: University of Michigan.

Whedon, M. B., & Shedd, P. (1989). Prediction and prevention of patient falls. *Image: The Journal of Nursing Scholarship, 21*(2), 108–114.

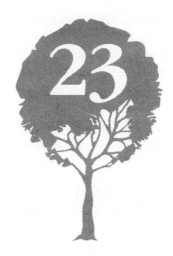

Practicing Environmental Accountability: A Mosaic of Meanings for Nursing

Carolyn L. Brown

N urses expressed their thoughtful commitment to environmental accountability for the nursing profession during
the conference represented in this book. After two days
of conference activities, small discussion groups met to explore
the meaning of nurses' accountability for the environment. Robert
and Phyllis Schultz, from the University of Washington, led one
group. Dianne LaCroix, from Victoria, Australia, led the other.*
Groups addressed these tasks:

*I am indebted to Phyllis and Robert Schultz and to Dianne LaCroix for leading
and summarizing the group discussions. The richness of this chapter attests to
their skill as group facilitators.

- Delineate how nurses might address environment as a domain of knowledge for the discipline of nursing.
- Highlight practical applications of environmental knowledge for the everyday work of nursing.
- Bring forward other issues or insights raised through participation in this environmental conference.

ADDRESSING ENVIRONMENT AS A DOMAIN OF NURSING KNOWLEDGE

In addressing environment as a domain of nursing knowledge, participants, uncovered a fundamental challenge for the profession. Like other humans, nurses face the challenge of letting go of old, comfortable assumptions about the nature of the world order. To embrace new assumptions raises the specter of uncertainty and heralds fundamental changes in the meaning of our lives. This can be scary. Embracing environmental accountability challenges the very core of our being, our identity. Nurses as individuals and as a professional group face the task of redefining their roles as healing professionals. One participant summarized by saying that ". . . environmental causes don't usually mobilize nurses unless it involves a physical sickness or a disaster." That nurses mobilize to heal what has already been diseased or injured lies at the heart of the definition of nursing knowledge. Such an assumption begs the questions of health promotion and disease prevention. Most nursing theories have given some attention to environment, but, except for Rogers (1970), Newman (1986), and Watson (1979, 1985), none has placed environment as central to nursing knowledge development. Assuming a healing role brings forward the basic question of who the recipient of nursing work should be. Could the environment be the focus of nurses' caring work?

From the discussion groups, these ideas about attending to environment in nursing knowledge development emerged:

- Environment is dynamic, living, and active. Environment is not a static void surrounding us as living beings.

- Environmental issues command attention from nurses on multiple levels of accountability, *now!*
- Environment is about nurses in dynamic interaction with new clients; Earth is to be included as a client.
- Environmental accountability calls for redefining nursing knowledge and expanding fundamental definitions of nursing.
- When nurses care for traditional clients and patients, including environment calls for an expanded definition of client. Statements from group discussion members graphically addressed this issue. For example, a participant stated: "Environment is more than the room or the building. What about how the patient's home environment contributes to illness? What flows behind the house, what does the patient breathe, ingest? . . . We are all members of community and we, as nurses, have to take some responsibility."
- Environmental accountability for nurses transcends traditional professional boundaries. Each nurse bears personal responsibility to have environmental accountability in personal life, as well as in the time spent at work. A participant stated, "We are the environment." As such, we are accountable for living that awareness.
- Environmental accountability includes open awareness of environmental interconnections in all practice decisions. Control of the environment may not be possible, and in many cases not desirable, but awareness allows informed choice among alternative approaches.
- Environmental responsibility extends to all areas of nursing practice and calls for flexible boundaries among specialty areas.
- Environmental accountability calls for expanded and flexible role definitions for nurses. Boundaries between realms of life—personal, spiritual, work, family—for nurses and those in need of nursing may also require reconceptualization. One discussion participant stated a case for ". . . extension of our knowledge in nursing. We should expand it and should start at an early age. Before, we were taught to separate ourselves from the environment and that is not how

it should be." Environmentally sensitive practice becomes a mandate pervading all nursing work roles, from traditional bedside nursing to the nurse entrepreneur, from case manager to corporate nurse executive.

• Reframing all nursing work to include its environmental context challenges each individual and the profession, *now* and as we move into the 21st century.

HIGHLIGHTING PRACTICAL APPLICATIONS OF EVERYDAY NURSING WORK

At the heart of practical applications lies the notion of rethinking, perhaps ReVisioning, such issues as control, advocacy, responsibility, and empowerment in environmentally accountable nursing relationships. Discussion group members made the following suggestions:

• Create practices where we develop respectful equity in all relationships.
• Include community assessments in practice and education. "The nurses in the acute care settings need to think of the hospital as a community and do a community assessment in that environment; . . . [in] that way, an institution would start looking at that organization as a whole within its context."
• Incorporate holism into nursing curricula.
• Observe the workplace to find the small actions that can greatly affect the environment. For example, a nurse working in the psychiatric area noticed the large number of small plastic medication bags labeled with patient identification data. Patients never touched them. Perhaps they could be recycled. Simply seeing our workplaces with a fresh eye, one sensitized with environmental awareness to see in a new way, creates opportunities for imaginative approaches to preserving the earth. Participants spoke of packaging supplies differently, checking fire extinguishers for safety of chemicals, recycling,

and finding ways to "recycle" leftover food in large organizations. These are simple actions having potential for starting an organizational level of environmental accountability. But, *someone* has to start it. Really seeing and assimilating the meaning of what assaults the senses begins the process.

- Use multiple approaches to heighten environmental accountability in organizations. One participant suggested, "Show them [administration] a financial benefit in an environmental issue. But that takes work, to find and assess the financial benefit."

- Reorganize the way care is provided. Providing more care outside the hospital may help decrease the vast amount of plastic trash. Recycle all plastic packing.

- Through purchasing committees, recommend use of products manufactured from recycled materials.

- Create awareness among work colleagues through your own efforts. Discuss environmental issues with colleagues.

- Recognize the amount of energy change requires. As one participant stated: "I really think that the thing we need to do more than anything is become aware and know that all the changes we are talking about are going to take tremendous social change. We all know how hard it is to make social change. I hope the planet will last long enough for us to do it. But if each of us changes one practice here and one practice there, and help one another to do that, we will make a difference. I know if I think that I have to change everything, I change nothing because it's too overwhelming, and I think I can't do it. So, perhaps we need to commit to change, and start small."

- Create model health care organizations operating according to environmental accountability.

- Ban disposable diapers in all health care facilities. Find or create a cost-efficient, safe alternative.

- For each choice made, ask, "Is it safe for the environment? How might this action do harm or good when it comes back to me, as it surely will?" Ask *many* questions!

- Be political. Understand and participate in political processes at all levels. For example, push for mass transportation, tax the right things (an example is to tax cigarettes to the maximum, but pay for and provide assistance for those who wish to stop smoking and need the help). Help legislators understand environmental accountability. Recommend they read Vice President Al Gore's book, *Earth in the Balance: Ecology and the Human Spirit* (1992).

- Encourage one another to be environmentally aware. Help one another reconnect with the earth.

- Encourage creativity. Learn what it is. Teach creativity in nursing education. Reward creative ideas, rather than squash them because they are different.

- Foster interdisciplinary dialogue about environmental issues. For example, form interdisciplinary environmental accountability committees in the workplace. Engage colleagues in casual conversation about the environment. When a colleague makes an unsound environmental decision, respectfully suggest a safer alternative.

- Create healthy and health-promoting workplace environments. Consider the air people breathe (how pure is it?), the chemicals used for cleaning, the odors people wear that may invade another's personal space, the food provided in the cafeteria, the pace of the work, the interpersonal environment, the way work is organized—to name just a few. Can healing take place in unhealthy settings? How many health care workers will become ill themselves by working in areas that encourage unhealthy practices or nurture unhealthy environments?

Through discussion, both groups identified a central concern for nurses thinking about taking on new challenges. Currently, the health care environment overwhelms nurses, depleting their personal and professional resources. Nurses are constantly asked to do more with less. If nurses see taking on the challenge of environmental accountability as just one more meaningless thing to do, one more task in an already overburdened work load, then the cause is lost. Environmental accountability extends to creating practice environments that nurture all health care providers and the environment. This quotation from a participant summarizes the concern: "I made another change, and another, and then when I thought I had done all the changing I could, someone else brings another idea, and I just couldn't do any more." The earlier suggestion, that each individual's single small actions have a large impact on the environment, is similar to the impact on individuals asked to do more. Multiple small demands on individuals, without finding ways to feed the energy system of those individuals, will eventually compromise their existence. They will burn out or become ill. To survive, they may fight any effort to further drain their personal resources, however well meaning the cause. Nurses who take on environmental challenges need to do so in ways that nurture themselves and others *now,* as they work for a sustainable planetary future.

OTHER ISSUES/INSIGHTS RAISED

As group participants reflected on their experiences with the conference program, a number expressed heightened consciousness of environmental issues. For example, one participant stated: "I am part of the environment and interconnected to the whole. If we see it this way, we see our roles. It becomes clear." Other ideas and insights identified included:

- Nursing and the environment have been disconnected. Environment has been viewed as a separate area of nursing knowledge. We need to start by teaching and living *connection.*
- Environment is not a single *something;* it becomes a different concept, depending on circumstances. Instead of being awed by the term, we need to use it flexibly, welcoming the diversity of definitions.
- To our peril, we and others often impose artificial limits on our responsibilities. The death knell for forward movement in nursing is the statement: "That's not nursing!" Let our practice be informed by nurses' taking on new challenges.

- We (all of us) are in a paradigm shift; this is an exciting time, because we are going to take big steps. We will *be there* when the universe turns over (Watson, 1993)!
- Both nursing and the environment are totally interrelated. Nurses create from that knowing!
- It's the jobs others create for nurses that interfere with what we want to do and be, as nurses. One person stated, "I love nursing; it's my job I hate!" We *can* take charge of creating our own work, sometimes by ourselves, sometimes in concert with others.

LOOKING BACK AND FORWARD

Discussion groups presented a collage of ideas for thinking about and enacting their commitment to environmental accountability. Participants were energized by the experience of finding a friendly forum for ideas. The diverse ideas in this chapter pose challenges to each of us. How might we redefine our practice? How might we take on the challenge of bringing environmental accountability into mainstream nursing through practice, research, and theory development? The ideas of the groups are simply listed here; they await fuller development by those willing to take on the challenge.

Everything recycles. Nothing is lost. Even the garbage in the land dump is recycled in a way we don't often think about. It forms noxious gases that come back to haunt us later. The question is whether the recycled products will harm those who live by the grace of Earth's generous provision. Barring a cosmic accident, the earth will persist, perhaps without life as we know it. If we do not take care of the planet, all life, as we know it, may cease to exist. New life forms may evolve, or earth could persist as a dead planet waiting for healing to birth new and friendlier entities.

Vice President Al Gore (1992) wisely recognizes the holographic nature of our existence on earth. Each of us can be likened to a part of a holograph where:

> . . . *the image becomes full and vivid only when that portion is combined with the rest of the [holographic] plate.*

Since I [Gore] first heard this phenomenon described, it has often struck me that it resembles the way each individual, like a single small part of a holographic plate, reflects, however faintly, a representation of the sum total of the values, choices, and assumptions that make up the society of which he or she is a part. (p. 11)

Change will happen in the whole of earth's fabric when each individual stops to take stock of who we are and how we enact what we profess to believe. ". . . [T]rue change is possible only when it begins inside the person who is advocating it" (Gore, 1992, p. 14). Thus, it seems to me, the wisdom from the discussion groups dictates the condition for change. For life-sustaining change to occur on this planet, each of us becomes a microcosmic representation of the whole of nursing and earth citizenship by living our commitment to environmental accountability.

REFERENCES

Gore, A. (1992). *Earth in the balance: Ecology and the human spirit.* New York: PLUME (Penguin).

Newman, M. (1986). *Health as expanding consciousness.* St. Louis, MO: Mosby.

Rogers, M. E. (1970). *An introduction to the theoretical basis of nursing.* Philadelphia: Davis.

Watson, J. (1979). *Nursing: The philosophy and science of caring.* Boston: Little, Brown.

Watson, J. (1985). *Nursing: Human science and human care.* Norwalk, CT: Appleton-Century-Crofts.

Watson, J. (1993, March). *Ecocaring as cosmology.* Keynote address presented at the conference on Expressions of Caring in Nursing: Exploring Our Environmental Connections, Boca Raton, FL.

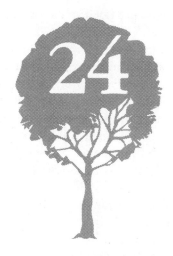

Endings and New Beginnings

Eleanor A. Schuster and Carolyn L. Brown

We bring this project to closure with a sense of awe and gratitude. Almost three years ago, we discussed in a faculty meeting that there "should be" an international conference specifically addressing nursing and the environment. The exact conclusion was: "If we don't do it, someone else will and why shouldn't that 'someone' be us?" From that time forward, the momentum increased, graced by the generosity, talents, enthusiasm, and tenacity of our colleagues, friends, and families. At that time, Florida Atlantic University had recently committed itself to becoming a center for environmental excellence. Allen Dines, President of Donnell-Kay, had provided generous funding to begin what was known as the FAU Environmental Initiative. The College of Nursing, encouraged by the institutional focus and direction as well as by strong administrative support from Dean Anne Boykin, was then poised to begin its special project. Iota Xi, FAU's local chapter of Sigma Theta Tau, nursing's honor society, shared the work and the financial commitment to mount an international conference within 10 months. (*Please note:* We strongly recommend at least 18 months to mount a major conference, based on our experience.) We learned early in the process that the effort had at least one precursor: The International Council of Nurses' International Nurses Day, 1990, with the theme, "Nurses and the Environment," May 12, 1990. In addition, our nurse colleagues in Australia, through the Australian Nursing Federation, were leaders in promoting and presenting a National Health and Ecology Conference in Melbourne, on March 25–26, 1993. This followed by several weeks our event in Boca Raton. We gratefully acknowledge now, as we did then, the immediate and ongoing assistance and encouragement of our Australian friends when they learned of our intent.

The coming together of an international group from nursing to experience and to deliberate about nursing's actual and potential accountability to the environment and for the environment was an aesthetically pleasing, scholarly event that nourished us in mind, body, and spirit. It also provided a clear challenge: this occasion must not remain only a nostalgic memory. Questions were raised: "What happens now?" "Where do we go from here?"

Responses to these questions are ongoing, and they vary in their level of visibility. For instance:

1. There was a call for follow-up conferences, and the possibility of a global coalition of nurses for the environment was mentioned. Australia, once again, is assuming leadership through an international conference slated for February, 1996.

2. Nursing and the environment, as a theme, is beginning to be evident in nursing scholarship. As an example, Dorothy Kleffel's doctoral dissertation is entitled, *The Environment: Alive, Whole, Interconnected and Interacting.*

3. A comprehensive instructional manual for implementing waste reduction and instituting recycling strategies in health care facilities has been co-authored by a nurse, Hollie Shaner (McRae, Shaner, & Bisson, 1993).

4. The book you are reading right now, strongly supported by the National League for Nursing, is one of several in development.

5. Specific directions for nursing curriculum changes are beginning to emerge. Betty Pennington's case study (Chapter 22) is an example of this movement.

One additional result was derived directly from the 1993 Boca Raton Conference: a group of Florida Atlantic University faculty, students, and administrators, in partnership with key community stakeholders, made a commitment to work toward establishing a Global Environmental Center for Healing and Health. To our knowledge, this is a first within a university's academic community. Two guiding questions for such a venture have been stated: (1) "How do we want to be cared for, now and into the future?" and (2) "How do we, as professionals, want to give care?" To gain specific direction and describe day-to-day steps in answering these two questions, a Future Search Conference entitled "Discovering Common Ground: The Future of Health, Healing and Environment" will convene in February 1995. A future search conference is a specific process through which invited representative stakeholders (in giving and receiving health care in our community) agree to come together to shape the future. In the environmental context, the future search process includes as stakeholders our air, soil, energy, and water, and includes life forms other than human. To date, the process has five characteristics that differentiate it from other healing and health centers:

1. Emphasis is on the interrelationships of health with environment;

2. There is focused bridge-building between and among professional disciplines;

3. There is a commitment to mainstream the effort within the university community;

4. There is reliance on the future search process, which includes *all* stakeholders, even those who dissent;

5. There is a commitment to serve the local communities while establishing and maintaining global networks.

At this time, other than having drafted a provisional mission statement, the work of the 9-member steering committee has been to provide a setting and enough financial support to allow the work and decision making of the stakeholders to occur through the future search conference process. The planners have become aware that the future search process is a healing modality in its own right. It is a way to form and welcome the future together, as a community, as contrasted to avoiding, fearing, or attempting to manipulate the future in isolated confusion.

All organizations exist within the environment. Each has an ethical responsibility to relate to that environment in ways that do no harm. That is the minimum standard. An even better standard is to assist the environment to heal itself. Like Florida Atlantic University, Barry University engages in an ongoing commitment to environmental concerns. In an effort to improve the quality of life for the neighborhood surrounding it, Barry University has started an initiative called "Pockets of Pride," under the leadership of its President, Sister Jeanne O'Laughlin, and her Executive Assistant, Sister Peggy Albert. By providing university resources to the surrounding community, Barry University works to assist the neighborhood to restore its environment and the homes of the residents in order to create a safe and healthy place for all who dwell there. Committed to service, Barry University also participates in volunteer Habitat for Humanity teams who provide housing within South Dade County. This initiative began as a response to Hurricane Andrew's devastation and has continued to serve the needs of that area. The Nursing Center of Barry University School of Nursing, through the collective efforts of faculty and students, coordinated by Associate Dean Patricia Munhall, provides health promotion and referral services to underserved families and children in the surrounding communities. Through this initiative, children learn to create healthy environments.

These are but a few of the efforts by two South Florida regional universities to enact environmental accountability. We know them best because they are our workplaces.

To show how endings can become new beginnings, here are some of the specific actions reported by participants in response to a four-month retrospective survey that asked a basic question: "What differences has this conference made in your everyday personal and professional lives?"

I am in touch again with my own deeply held beliefs about our natural world.

I am networking with those of like mind from the conference, and have an increased awareness of the importance of networking.

I asked to get on our environmental committee at our hospital.

I am working with some other nurses at our hospital to form a Nursing Environmental Task Force.

I have cemented a personal philosophy of caring in all *settings.*

I have entered a nonnursing Master's program to further my beliefs in a holistic model of health and caring.

I am more aware of the interconnecting web of all life.

I am exploring the ecological life-style of voluntary simplicity in my own life.

Holistic feminism in nursing is important to me, and I intend to look for these elements in my search for doctoral programs.

I reflect each evening on what I have done that day to protect the environment and how I plan to live day-by-day.

There was almost a 60% return rate of the follow-up questionnaire, indicating to us, as conference coordinators, a high level of personal interest and investment in the conference experience and its ramifications for daily living.

THE FUTURE

We believe the future is open. We believe we have options, in our private and professional lives, of who and how we want to be in the world. We invite each reader to consider giving priority to day-to-day choices that will enlarge and enrich nursing's environmental connections and refine our sense of accountability.

We think it fitting to close this book by honoring an early dweller of this land, the Osage woman, who was responsible for planting, cultivating, and harvesting corn. The poem we selected (La Flesche, 1921) is unusual because it places a mark of human identity at the sacred center of its world. Like many other songs and chants, it uses repetition as a way of calling forth order into the world.

An Osage Woman's Initiation Song

I have made a footprint, a sacred one.
I have made a footprint, through it the blades push upward.
I have made a footprint, through it the blades radiate.
I have made a footprint, over it the blades float in the wind.
I have made a footprint, over it the blossoms lie grey.
I have made a footprint, smoke arises from my house.
I have made a footprint, there is cheer in my house.
I have made a footprint, I live in the light of day.

PERSONAL STATEMENT (ELEANOR SCHUSTER)

I grew up out-of-doors, first on Florida's eastern shores, embraced by sun, surf, and sand; then in the West, mainly in Arizona, where I learned to hear "the sound of silence." In my mind's eye, I can still stand in the company of the monument rock sentinels and sacred mesas of Navajo and Hopi country. My friends and playmates were the trees, plants, shells, and animals, as well as other children.

Within the past decade or so, I have realized with increasing clarity that the only thing we humans *have,* as a gift in return, is *the way we live our lives.* Everything else has been given us—our being, our gifts and talents, material goods, food, shelter, friendships, and more. Our challenge as humans is to learn to reciprocate the giving. Our path is to dance, sing, and celebrate the cosmos, and, when we leave, hope that the echo of our songs remains.

REFERENCES

La Flesche, F. (1921). *The Osage tribe,* vol. I, 36th annual report, Bureau of American Ethnology, Washington, DC.

McRae, G., Shaner, H., & Bisson, C. L. (1993). *An ounce of prevention: Waste reduction strategies for health care facilities.* Chicago: American Hospital Association.

DATE DUE

APR 1 0 '01			